Men's Health

Life Improvement Guides™

Stronger Faster

Workday Workouts That
Build Maximum Muscle
in Minimum Time

by Brian Paul Kaufman, Sid Kirchheimer,
and the Editors of **Men'sHealth** Books

Rodale Press, Inc.
Emmaus, Pennsylvania

Other titles in the *Men's Health Life Improvement Guides* series:

Command Respect	*Good Loving*	*Stress Blasters*
Death Defiers	*Maximum Style*	*Symptom Solver*
Fight Fat	*Powerfully Fit*	*Vitamin Vitality*
Food Smart	*Sex Secrets*	

Library of Congress Cataloging-in-Publication Data

Kaufman, Brian, 1961–
    Stronger faster : workday workouts that build maximum muscle in minimum time / by Brian Paul Kaufman, Sid Kirchheimer, and the editors of Men's Health Books.
       p.   cm. — (Men's health life improvement guides)
    Includes index.
    ISBN 0–87596–359–5 paperback
    1. Physical fitness for men. 2. Exercise for men. I. Kirchheimer, Sid. II. Men's Health Books. III. Title. IV. Series.
GV482.5.K38 1997
613.7'0449—dc21
                                                   96–48687

Distributed in the book trade by St. Martin's Press

  4 6 8 10 9 7 5 3   paperback

—— OUR PURPOSE ——

"We inspire and enable people to improve their lives and the world around them."

Stronger Faster Editorial Staff

Senior Managing Editor: **Neil Wertheimer**

Senior Editor: **Jack Croft**

Writers: **Brian Paul Kaufman, Sid Kirchheimer, Alisa Bauman, Perry Garfinkel, Stephen C. George, Wendy Wetherbee**

Contributing Writers: **Kelly Elizabeth Coffey, Jane Unger Hahn**

Researchers and Fact Checkers: **Sally A. Reith, Jennifer Barefoot, Kelly Elizabeth Coffey, Raymond M. Di Cecco, Jane Unger Hahn, Sarah Wolfgang Heffner, Margo Trott**

Copy Editors: **Amy K. Kovalski, David R. Umla**

Series Art Director: **Charles Beasley**

Book Designer: **Thomas P. Aczel**

Cover Designer: **Charles Beasley**

Cover Photographer: **Mitch Mandel**

Photo Editor: **Susan Pollack**

Illustrators: **Thomas P. Aczel, Mark Matcho**

Studio Manager: **Stefano Carbini**

Technical Artists: **J. Andrew Brubaker, Mary Brundage**

Manufacturing Coordinator: **Melinda B. Rizzo**

Office Staff: **Roberta Mulliner, Julie Kehs, Bernadette Sauerwine, Mary Lou Stephen**

Rodale Health and Fitness Books

Vice-President and Editorial Director: **Debora T. Yost**

Design and Production Director: **Michael Ward**

Research Manager: **Ann Gossy Yermish**

Copy Manager: **Lisa D. Andruscavage**

Book Manufacturing Director: **Helen Clogston**

Photo Credits

Cover and all photographs by **Mitch Mandel** except those listed below.

Page 136: **Craig Blankenhorn**

Page 138: **Eric Crossan**

Page 140: **Michael Ahearn**

Page 142: **Courtesy of Northwestern University**

Page 144: **Courtesy of Spyglass, Inc.**

Page 146: **Jim Block**

Contents

Part Four

Getting the Edge

Part Five

Real-Life Scenarios

Quest for the Best

You Can Do It!

Male Makeovers

Introduction

The Active Life

The Scottish playwright J. M. Barrie, whose best-known work, *Peter Pan*, chronicles the adventures of a boy who refuses to grow up, once remarked: "It is not real work unless you would rather be doing something else."

That might explain the word *work* in workouts. For too many guys, exercise is something to be endured, not enjoyed. We set aside a defined amount of time—20 minutes, half an hour, 45 minutes, an hour—and spend it working out. Day in and day out, we work. And we work out. And if we're honest, most of the time we'd rather be doing something else.

Perhaps we have the whole notion of exercise wrong. We need to stop thinking of fitness in terms of whether we got to the gym three times last week. Rather, think of fitness as a lifestyle that touches on everything we do.

Just as our work life helps define who we are, so does our fitness life. This is not to say that a man is defined solely by his job (or, as we're suggesting, his activity level). But there is still something to be said for the justifiable pride a man can take in a job well done.

The same goes for a body well done. And it seems that men are starting to make the connection. One survey of men in their thirties and forties found that 67 percent cited being healthy and fit as a key factor in their personal definition of success.

But what does it mean to be healthy and fit? Surely, it's more than that half-hour spent in the gym or running on the roads. The answer can be found in the hundreds of small choices we make every day. Do you smack the snooze button on the alarm clock, or do you get up in time to eat a healthy breakfast and do a few stretches before heading off to work? When you arrive at the office, do you park as close to the building as possible or in the farthest lot to get in a brisk walk? If your office is on the third floor, do you take the stairs or the elevator?

Extend that to home. Do you climb trees with your kids or watch videos with them? Do you hire the neighbor's kid to cut the lawn while you watch the NCAA game of the week, or do you do it yourself? Is your hobby bicycling or the Internet?

Our message: The active life isn't defined by the block of time you set aside to exercise each day (although that certainly is an important part of the fitness equation). It's defined by all those other little things you probably don't even think about.

Which brings us to this book. *Stronger Faster* is jam-packed with tips and programs on how to get as much exercise as you can into a busy day. Weight lifting, stretching, running, bicycling—we'll show you how to do all those and more as efficiently and effectively as possible. We even go so far as to tell you how to pack a lunch, take a shower, and fill your gym bag in ways that maximize your time for exercise and active fun.

But underlying the entire book is this key message: Fitness is a lifestyle, not three visits to the gym a week. It's about making moment-to-moment choices that maximize health, strength, and energy. It's choosing to go through life with vigor, be it bounding up the stairs at work or bounding up the mountainside with your dog.

And don't be surprised if, while you're slaving away at the office, you suddenly realize that the something else you'd rather be doing is working out. Some guys never grow up.

Neil Wertheimer
Senior Managing Editor, *Men's Health* Books

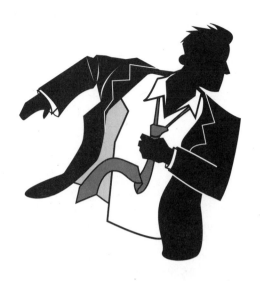

Part One

Working In the Workouts

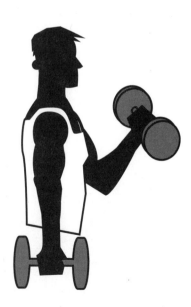

Finding Time for Fitness

Make an Investment in Your Future

Ever so slowly, the sun clears the horizon, signaling the start of another workday. Somewhere, a rooster crows. The missus puts on a pot of coffee and opens the kitchen curtains to let in the streaky morning light. Bacon sizzles. The radio crackles.

Pastoral daybreak. It's a quaint symbol of a different world, one that's simple and honest and orderly.

Then there's *our* lives.

The frenetic pace of the workplace doesn't wait for some plodding celestial ball or loud-mouthed farm animal anymore. The world of commerce hurls forward 24 hours a day, seven days a week. It is always there, gnawing at our brains, eating at our time. According to a study by phone giant MCI, more than half of all Americans now say they believe that the distinction between work and personal time has blurred.

Mega-mergers. Superstores. Surging start-up companies. The global marketplace. Stock offerings. Home-based businesses. The World Wide Web. Corporate downsizing. Employee buyouts. This is our lives, men, and we had best learn to live with it.

Most men make an uneasy peace with their frenetic existences. But we have a secret. We know a way to cope with the weight of living far better than you could ever imagine. This method gives you stamina, energy, a sharper mind, a competitive edge, a

stress-resilient body. The time you invest in this method you'll get back many times over.

Our secret?

Exercise. The ultimate capitalist's tool.

A Shrewd Investment

Some of the busiest and most successful folks on the planet have come to look at their workouts not as a chore or an indulgence, but as an important investment in their future.

"As a result of sacrificing the 30 to 60 minutes five days a week necessary for me to achieve physical fitness, I'm able to sustain high productivity for four or more hours each day," says Zig Ziglar, motivational speaker and author of the audiocassettes *Goals: Setting and Achieving Them on Schedule.* "So I invest one hour and get back a minimum of four hours top performance—and most of the time, considerably more than that. I don't have to find time under those circumstances. I schedule the time, utilize that time, and get my return on investment immediately, plus ensuring a higher quality of life, all of my life."

James M. Rippe, M.D., associate professor of medicine at Tufts University School of Medicine in Boston and author of *Fit over Forty,* concurs: "The main benefit I get out of my exercise program is stress reduction. So literally, the busier I am, the more important for me it is to work out."

And this is just stretching the benefits of exercise to the work world. Fitness, as you 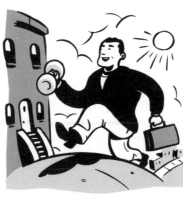 know, touches on *every* aspect of your life. With exercise, you'll:

• Look and feel better

• Cut your risk of deadly diseases, including heart problems and diabetes

• Have better sex and even prevent impotence

• Meet new people, develop friendships, or maybe even find your future mate

• Boost your self-confidence many times over

Who Knows Where the Time Goes?

If there's little doubt about the benefits of working out—especially for us working stiffs—why aren't more of us doing it?

Lifestyle studies provide some clues. According to a comprehensive study ominously called the Americans' Use of Time Project, men have an average of 40 hours of free time a week—nearly five hours of leisure each Monday through Friday, seven hours on Saturday, and eight hours on Sunday.

"Today the 40-hour workweek is balanced by the 40-hour play week," says John P. Robinson, Ph.D., professor of sociology at the University of Maryland in College Park and director of the project. "It may be hard to believe, but that's about seven hours more free time than we had two decades ago."

Each year, The NPD Group, a consumer marketing research firm in Rosemont, Illinois, has 3,000 people from across the country—1,500 men and 1,500 women between the ages of 18 and 90 and representing all economic classes—complete a diary of what they do every hour for 24 hours. And although there have been some slight changes, vice-president Harry Balzer reports that the data seem to have held steady over the past four years.

The result is that sleep takes the largest chunk of our time: 7 hours and 25 minutes a day. Work-related activities like grooming and commuting and work itself take up the next biggest block: 4 hours and 42 minutes. (Because this number is averaged over seven days and includes people who don't work, it's a little misleading. Working adults who filled out the diary actually said they worked 7.5 hours a day.)

However, that's not to say that a lot of us aren't working longer and harder than ever before. Remember, the 7.5-hour workday was only an average. Between 1973 and 1993, the number of men working 49 hours a week or more had increased from 23.9 percent to 29.2 percent, according to the Division of Labor Force Statistics of the U.S. Bureau of Labor Statistics.

But in The NPD Group time survey, entertainment—things like watching TV and videos, listening to music, reading, or visiting friends—came in third. Total time spent per day on entertainment was 4 hours and 23 minutes, says Balzer.

Now before you claim to be working your way down the *New York Times* best-seller's list, the folks at Nielson Media Research, the New York–based organization that tracks TV viewing habits, report that average daily viewing for men 18 and older is 3 hours and 52 minutes.

On the other hand, The NPD Group's study found that, on average, people spend just 15 minutes each day exercising, Balzer says.

And yet a study for the President's Council on Physical Fitness and Sports found that 42 percent of those who don't exercise say that they don't have enough time, says Mary Ann Hill, director of communications for the President's Council on Physical Fitness and Sports in Washington, D.C.

"Some people say, 'I'm not going to work out today because I don't have a whole hour to take 10 minutes to walk to the gym and change my clothes and work out for 35 minutes and take a shower and come back.' But you don't need a whole hour every day. You could walk briskly for 20 minutes if that's all the time you have. Or 10 minutes. Find some time for fitness and use it," Hill says.

Dr. Rippe agrees. "Many people haven't figured out how to fit exercise into their life. They haven't prioritized it. They don't understand that you can fit it in different ways, that you can accumulate exercise rather than having to do it at one session. But the biggest barrier that the non-exerciser has to overcome is his perception that he doesn't have time. It's not the reality that he doesn't have time. It's his perception that he doesn't have time."

Over the course of this book, we're going to show you hundreds of ways to reclaim your time so that you can work out. And we'll also share plenty of ways to get more out of your workout. A new workout day has dawned.

How Healthy Are You?

Put Yourself to the Test

All Tim Klooster had to do to get another beer when he was atop his Sears riding lawn mower was to raise an empty and shake it.

"The kids would see that and run and get me another one," Klooster says. "It was a big lawn—a three- or four-beer job."

Of course, that was 50 pounds ago. Before he bagged his 1½-packs-a-day smoking habit. Before Klooster took part in an employee wellness program at Steelcase, the world's largest manufacturer of office furniture.

Today, the 39-year-old Grand Rapids, Michigan, resident works out two hours every other day and runs marathons in his spare time. Heck, he even married the exercise physiologist who works in the Steelcase wellness center. They first got to know each other when she was giving him a fitness test. "It changed my life, no doubt about it," he says.

Such dramatic stories seem contrived— like a weight-loss marketer's dream. Yet in workplaces and gyms and homes around the country, something amazing is happening. Men who, until now, would just as soon smoke, eat, drink, and lounge their way to an early grave are discovering that a few simple lifestyle changes can make life-altering improvements in their health and fitness.

"Of course, we can't promise or guarantee anything, but if you make an effort to improve or to practice recommended lifestyle behaviors, it's safe to say that you'll have a higher probability of overall general health and a

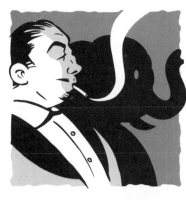

reduced chance of disease and illness," says Elaine Schnueringer, research associate in the University of Michigan's Health Management Research Center in Ann Arbor.

Research shows that exercise plays an unparalleled role in health improvement. One massive study by the famed Cooper Institute for Aerobic Research in Dallas found that even smokers with high blood pressure and cholesterol who are in good aerobic shape tend to live longer than people who don't exercise or smoke. Yet the evidence is clear: Exercise is only part of the solution.

There are much more elaborate health tests—ones that require lots of tubes and electrodes and phalanxes of specialists to interpret the data. But the self-exam found on the opposite page—developed by Kenneth Blanchard, Ph.D.; D. W. Edington, Ph.D.; and Marjorie Blanchard, Ph.D., at the University of Michigan's Health Management Research Center—is a quick way to help you understand the variety of factors that can contribute to good or poor health.

At least that's what Steelcase employees discovered after the company implemented dozens of educational and incentive programs in the 1980s to help them shed unhealthy habits and get fit.

As a result, University of Michigan researchers for the first time in a large-scale study documented the link between lifestyle behaviors and the reduced need for medical care.

In an effort that included programs for stopping smoking and substance abuse, one-on-one counseling, and increasing physical activity— from fun runs to negotiating cheaper rates at area health clubs—the number of employees with high cholesterol dropped from 20 percent to 13 percent over a five-year period. Company medical costs and absenteeism dropped. But more important, lives were changed. Lives like Tim Klooster's.

Look at Your Life

Statement	Yes	No
1. *I love my job most of the time.*	☐	☐
2. *I take good safety precautions such as using a seat belt in a moving vehicle.*	☐	☐
3. *I am within five pounds of my ideal weight.*	☐	☐
4. *I know three methods to reduce stress that do not include the use of drugs or alcohol.*	☐	☐
5. *I do not smoke.*	☐	☐
6. *I sleep six to eight hours each night and wake up refreshed.*	☐	☐
7. *I engage in regular physical activity at least three times per week (including sustained physical exertion for 20 to 30 minutes, that is, walking briskly, running, swimming, biking, plus stretching and flexibility activities).*	☐	☐
8. *I have seven or fewer alcoholic drinks per week.*	☐	☐
9. *I know my blood pressure and cholesterol.*	☐	☐
10. *I follow sensible eating habits (eat breakfast daily; limit salt, sugar, and fats; limit eggs, whole milk, breakfast meats, cheese, and red meats; eat adequate fiber).*	☐	☐
11. *I have a good social support system.*	☐	☐
12. *I maintain a positive mental attitude.*	☐	☐

Scoring

Give yourself one point for every "Yes" checked.

- *0–6*   *Your behaviors may be hazardous to your lifestyle.*
- *7–9*   *You are on the positive side.*
- *10–12*   *Congratulations! You're living life at its best.*

What It Means

If you are scoring in the top category, you are managing your life for the highest return and highest quality of life. Behavioral change is not easy—if you are interested in changing any of your "no" answers to "yes," pick an easy one to begin. After you succeed, pick another one.

The Science of Building Muscle

Becoming a Lean Machine

Pick up any bodybuilding magazine, and if you can get past the women in bikinis who look like they could bench-press a small Chevy, you can't help but notice the mind-boggling number of programs, techniques, gizmos, powders, and pills touted for building muscle. "Whey Protein: The Magic Muscle Builder," screams one headline. "Blast your Biceps for Maximum Peak and Definition," says another. "Insulin Surge: The Key to Muscle Growth."

And since the guys pictured in those magazines are huge—almost as big as the women, in fact—you're left to wonder: Which magic formula am I, Mr. Time Crunch, supposed to use if I just want to add an inch or two to my arms or chest?

There is a formula, but there's nothing magic about it and it doesn't come in any bottle. Once you understand the basic principles of training, nutrition, and recovery, it's just a matter of fine-tuning them to meet your body's needs before you start filling out your suits with brand new muscle. Best of all, it doesn't take much time in the gym either— about an hour every other day at the most— and your muscles begin to grow almost immediately.

"A neophyte, a new weight lifter, can be on the worst workout routine in the world, and he will probably still make tremendous gains because it's such a new experience for his muscles," says Bob Lefavi, Ph.D., a sports nutrition and strength-training specialist at Armstrong Atlantic State University in Savannah, Georgia, and the 1990

International Federation of Bodybuilding North American bantamweight bodybuilding champion. "Even guys who have been spending too much time in the gym will see gains if they alter their programs."

Building muscle naturally offers nothing but benefits. For one thing, research shows that adding lean body mass acts as a built-in fat burner. In fact, for every pound of muscle you gain, your resting metabolic rate goes up 50 calories a day.

"When people begin replacing their body fat with lean muscle, their body tends to become a much more efficient machine," says Bob Goldman, D.O., Ph.D., chairman of the American Academy of Anti-Aging Medicine and president of the National Academy of Sports Medicine in Chicago.

There's also increasing evidence that building muscle the natural way helps ward off, and even reverse, the effects of degenerative diseases like arthritis. Researchers have found that people with arthritis who are placed on strength-training programs are stronger, have fewer symptoms, have increased range of motion, and lose weight, Dr. Goldman says.

Twitch Way Do You Go?

Bulging biceps and chiseled pectorals get all the attention, but those show muscles are just two of the 215 pairs of skeletal muscles found in your body—regardless of whether you've ever lifted weights. Some are tiny, like the nine that control movement in your thumb. Others can be huge. When fully developed, your latissimus dorsi, located on either side of your back and torso, can give you a V-shape that would make the Caped Crusader jealous.

Like a tightly woven rope, each muscle is composed of fibers—microscopic strands ranging in length from a few millimeters to those running the length of your thigh. Roughly divided into fast-twitch and slow-twitch fibers, each has a specific purpose. When you think fast-twitch, think force and bulk—they're the ones at work when someone's hammering out a set of monster bench presses or sprinting to victory. Slow-twitch muscle fibers provide the aerobic endurance for you to keep your leg muscles pumping on a stair-climber.

Although most of us are born with an equal amount of both fast- and slow-twitch fibers, there's little doubt that some folks are literally built for building muscle. "Look at (former professional football and baseball star) Bo Jackson. You probably won't see him running a marathon. He's a strength and power athlete, born with a far greater proportion of fast-twitch muscle fibers than the average person. So Jackson is more muscular than, let's suppose, a fraternal twin of his who did not have that high a percentage of fast-twitch fibers," Dr. Lefavi says.

But how does any muscle fiber, fast- or slow-twitch, get bigger? Quite simply, the potential for building muscle begins when you challenge your muscles in a new or different way—whether it's with push-ups, dumbbell curls, a long run or bike ride, swinging golf clubs for the first time in six months, or, heck, maybe even 1 out of every 1,000 workout gadgets advertised on late-night cable TV.

Here's why. Just as a matter of course, your muscles break down every 7 to 15 days, replacing old cells and doing some general housekeeping. But when you stress your muscles through weight training or some other form of resistance exercise, the cells that make up the muscle fibers actually break down faster. "It's like what happens when you walk on the beach," Dr. Lefavi says. "If you haven't been there in a while, by virtue of the fact that your heel sinks into the sand, that challenges your

Be a Vary Strong Guy

If you look around the gym, it's easy to spot the guys who have fallen into a rut. They look no different than they did six months ago.

"Show me a guy who hasn't changed his routine for a while and I'll show you a guy who hasn't changed his physique in a while either," says Armstrong Atlantic State University's Dr. Bob Lefavi.

As a result, most experts suggest changing your routine every three months to keep your muscles growing. Consider switching to a low-rep strength-training program for a few months. Or break your routine into two parts, training your upper body one day and lower body the next. Or you may not even want to wait that long.

"Some days you may feel like you have been under a lot of stress, and you just don't want to get under any heavy weight. Great. That's a perfect day to throw some light weights on the bar and burn out a bunch of reps. Using a 15-rep max or 20-rep max is a great variation. That will really throw something different at your muscles and force them to grow. That's what it's all about," Dr. Lefavi says.

calf muscles in a new way. And you can feel it the next day—you're sore. Or you play softball over the weekend for the first time in 10 years, and on Monday you feel all these muscles in your back and your shoulders that you forgot you had."

Although the actual cause of that soreness sparks heated debate at most sports medicine conferences, the prevailing view suggests that intense exercise causes both microscopic tears in the muscle and the breakdown of protein in the muscle.

But your muscles don't take the abuse lying down. "It's as if the muscle cell says, 'You've given me a stress that I'm not accustomed to and you've injured me, and I don't ever want to go through that injury again. So this time, I'm not going to repair myself to where I was. I'm going to repair myself a little bit better and a little bit bigger so that the next time you give me this stress, I won't have to go through it again.' And that's how growth occurs," Dr. Lefavi says.

Feeding Your Muscles

If resistance exercise gets your muscle's attention, it still needs several things to fulfill its vow to rebuild bigger and stronger than ever. Among them is proper nutrition. Just what constitutes proper nutrition for muscle building is another controversial area—witness the endless flood of products that suggest they can help you pack on the muscular pounds.

While most experts remain skeptical of such claims for all but a few products, there seems to be general agreement that your intake of protein and total calories should increase if you want to add lean body mass. "The bottom line is this: If you're not consuming enough energy, then you are going to be in trouble either maintaining or building muscle," says Peter Lemon, Ph.D., director of the Department of Applied Physiology at Kent State University in Kent, Ohio. "So priority number one has to be energy."

Even for those of us who were born without that all-important math gene, the equation is simple. If you don't eat enough to replace the calories that your body is burning off when you're weight training, you'll actually lose weight and muscle mass. But figuring out how much to eat is a little trickier. "In some studies of very good weight lifters, their energy intake was approximately double. But if you're not training quite as hard, you obviously won't need as much," says Dr. Lemon.

Generally, Dr. Lemon recommends eating about 40 calories per kilogram of body weight when trying to build muscle. That means that the average 170-pound man might need to eat roughly 3,100 calories a day. A 230-pounder should knock back about

4,200 calories a day or more.

But unfortunately for pork rind–lovers, not just any calories will do. You'll need to make sure that you're eating between 1.4 and 1.8 grams of protein for every kilogram of body weight. That translates into about 123 grams of protein for a 170-pound man and about 167 grams for a 230-pound guy. (Just to give you an idea, three ounces of albacore tuna packs 25.1 grams of protein, a three-ounce chicken breast has 26.7 grams, and an eight-ounce glass of 2% low-fat milk contains 8.1 grams.) Why protein? Although more research needs to be done, it's thought that once the protein has been broken down in your blood into amino acids, your muscle cells use them to rebuild.

Newly fortified, the muscle fiber literally begins to grow in preparation for the next workout assault. And before long, bigger fibers mean bigger muscles. "At one time we thought that you might be splitting the fibers, in essence, creating new ones, but now we're convinced that you're just making the old ones larger," Dr. Goldman says.

Dr. Lemon explains: "If you aren't getting enough amino acids in your diet, then you'll pull those from other areas of the body—you'll actually be degrading some protein sources like muscle to build others. Obviously, you don't want to be doing that if you're trying to build muscle mass."

But don't rush out and snatch up all the canned tuna fish at your local grocery store just yet. Most guys eat that much protein during the day anyway. Do the math first and then make a shopping trip if you have to.

Aside from some research that suggests that your calcium and magnesium needs might increase while you're resistance training, there still isn't hard evidence to support higher vitamin and mineral requirements for those trying to build muscle. At least not yet.

"I think that in due course some of these nutrients will be shown to be higher. And it makes sense. Some of these nutrients are involved in processes rapidly accelerated by exercise. And let's not forget that the Daily Values have been established based on people who, if not totally sedentary, are at least mostly sedentary. And they are being applied to people who train at very intense levels," Dr. Lemon says. Although more research needs to be done, a substance that has considerable promise as a muscle builder is creatine, he says.

So once you're training and eating right, how much muscle can you expect to build? "Over a six-week period we see anywhere from four to five pounds of muscle. So on average you might get a pound a week of muscle mass. But obviously, if you eat too much, you can put on fat at the same time," says Dr. Lemon.

Another factor that determines muscle growth is your testosterone level, the uniquely male hormone that helps stimulate muscle growth. More testosterone usually means more muscle mass—the same reason that many bodybuilders take steroids. If your testosterone level is high, it's likely that you'll be able to pack on the beef more quickly than the guy down the block who works out just as hard but has low testosterone. Even rest—giving your muscles time to rebuild—plays a role. Experts say that it takes between 48 and 72 hours for your muscles to recover from a workout.

But there's more to building muscle than just eating right and showing up at the gym—you have to know what to do when you're there.

Ready, Set, Superset

In your quest for speed and variety in your weight-training program, try two techniques used by more advanced lifters: supersets and tri-sets.

To do a superset, simply perform one exercise—a barbell curl, for example—rest for about 30 seconds, and then exercise the opposing muscle, in this case, your triceps, according to Bill Pearl of Phoenix, Oregon, former Mr. Universe and author of *Getting Stronger*. After that set, wait about one minute and then repeat.

"If you're trying to gain more mass, 8 to 10 reps would be a good idea; but if you're trying to drop weight, it may not be a bad idea to keep the reps anywhere from 12 to 14 and maybe as high as 20—depending on what you are attempting to do with your body," Pearl says. If you're trying to gain muscle but are crunched for time, two supersets for each muscle you're training that day should suffice, he says.

A tri-set is a group of three exercises, each done after the other—again with limited rest in between. Tri-sets can be used to work three different muscle groups, different areas of the same muscle from three different angles, or the same area of a muscle, says Pearl.

But be careful. Like any other weight-training programs, supersets and tri-sets can cause injury if not performed properly. "You don't want to go to one exercise, do the exercise, throw the weights down, and run back again," Pearl says.

Mastering the Movement

Judging from the incredible, vein-laced bulks pictured in most bodybuilding magazines, you'd get the impression that you have to hoist massive weights for hours on end to build muscle.

Thankfully, for the busy guy who has a life and wants to look like he works out, it's not so. "Those folks who are training intensely and consistently for 1½ to 2 hours are either overtraining or taking enough drugs to kill a cow," Dr. Lefavi says. "I've been around gyms and bodybuilding long enough to say that without maligning anyone. That's just the way it is."

Instead, most experts suggest choosing a core group of exercises for your chest, back, arms, shoulders, abdominals, and legs that you perform, at most, three times a week—and preferably, just twice. Beginners should perform one or two sets per exercise. More advanced lifters should do three or four sets per exercise—and no more.

It's also best that you pick a weight that you can lift for no more than 8 to 12 repetitions. "Typically with women, we tell them to pick a weight that they can only do for 12 reps maximum, and they pick a weight they can do for 50 reps and stop at 10. By the same token, the average guy picks a weight that he can do 4 reps with, and I have to help him with 6 more. Go figure," Dr. Lefavi says.

Simply put, a 12-rep max is a weight that you can lift for 12 repetitions, but not even one more.

Although training with heavier weights for lower reps seems to produce the biggest strength and power gains, 8 to 12 reps maximum seems to build muscle faster in most people, says Dr. Lefavi. But if you're a beginner, you'll be thrilled to know that for the first three months, you're bound to see increases in both.

Some of those strength gains come as a result of what experts call neuromuscular learning. Just figuring out how to correctly perform a squat or bench press in a "biomechanically efficient pattern" takes skill, says Dr. Lefavi. "It's not a whole lot different from learning to swing a golf club. You have to swing it just the right way, in just the right biomechanical pattern. Meanwhile, intramuscular changes start taking place—like the amino acid accumulation and synthesis going on within the muscle cells that cause muscle growth. Let's put it this way, if you've just started weight training three months ago and don't notice an enhancement of your strength or musculature, you're doing something wrong."

One common error made by beginners that can actually prevent growth is overtraining. Enthusiasm for your new muscle building routine is fine, but when that translates into pitching a tent near the squat rack, you're probably just holding yourself back.

"There's no body part that I know of that really needs to be trained from more than three angles, in other words, more than three exercises," says Dr. Lefavi. "And I would say that for the smaller singular-joint muscles, like the biceps or traps or forearms, you don't need to do more than one or two exercises."

Another way to make sure that you don't overtrain is watching the clock between sets. The good news for guys on the go is that experts don't want you to spend more than an hour in the gym. In fact, you may want to take your exit cue from any elite, non-steroid-using weight lifter or bodybuilder in your gym—that's when *they'll* be hitting the door.

"Spend the first 15 minutes warming up. Ride a stationary bike to get a little cardiovascular exercise in and help get the inner temperature of your muscles up. And then you'll have time to do a couple sets per exercise and a couple exercises per body part," says Dr. Lefavi. "You want to fully tax the muscles in a comprehensive and rapid fashion so that within a 35- to 40-minute period, you're done with your workout."

How do you know whether you're overtraining? If your muscles are still sore heading into your next training session, your muscles have not completely recovered. "Recovery is a really tricky area, but so far this is one of the best gauges we have," Dr. Lefavi says. "We think that most muscles are able to repair themselves within two to three days when they've been trained with average intensity. But when someone is just starting out, it could be five to six days before a muscle is ready to be stimulated again." How do you know? The answer is, you can't. But if you're still sore, that's a good indication that you need to hold off, he says.

A Strength-Training Primer

Time Is on Your Side

You tell yourself that the important thing is just getting to the gym to lift. How much you can bench-press doesn't really matter, you say.

And sometimes, you almost believe it. But let's be truthful, men. When it's your turn to bench, it would do wonders for your self-esteem if you had to ask the guys to throw on a couple more 45-pound plates—rather than sheepishly asking them to take them off.

Make no mistake, anyone who's been lifting for a while will tell you that getting stronger is hard work that takes time—with success often measured in years. But the inherent principles of strength training—low reps with heavy weights—may actually serve you better physically and emotionally during particularly busy and stressful times than elaborate cross-training and other workout programs.

In fact, research shows that when it comes to building Samsonlike strength, two to three months of short but intense training sessions are best—perfect for a busy guy with a life. Not only that, but power-lifting movements such as squats and cleans exercise several muscle groups simultaneously, also helping cut training time. And if you've been stuck in a training rut, strength training may very well blast you to another round of size and strength increases.

"That's why athletes like power lifters and Olympic shot-putters go through various training phases where they will develop muscle mass, and then

they will try to peak their ability to demonstrate that strength by lifting heavier weights. Same principle," says Steven Fleck, Ph.D., former head of the physical conditioning program for the U.S. Olympic program and a sports physiologist in Silverthorne, Colorado.

Man versus Machine

If you asked most strength coaches to choose between training in one of those mauve-carpeted "fitness studios" adorned with chrome-plated machines or a room containing only a pair of concrete blocks and a pipe, most would probably choose the latter. And not because they're old-fashioned. Free weights simply test your muscles in ways that many machines can't.

"People concerned with 'fitness' tend to use machines that allow them to perform what we call single-joint exercises—things like leg extensions and bicep curls," says Boyd Epley, director of athletic performance and assistant athletic director at the University of Nebraska in Lincoln. "And that's fine, but if you really want to gain strength, training with free weights helps you develop your synergistic muscles—the muscles that support the bones of the muscles that you are trying to train. And that's a big plus that you can't get any other way."

Consider the squat. "When you're doing a squat, you are working your legs," Epley says. "But if your stomach and lower back

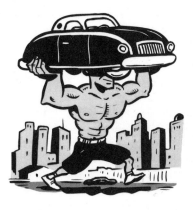

don't contract isometrically and become stabilizers, you don't get the proper development of your legs. These synergistic muscles do their job so that the legs can move correctly and get the benefit."

In fact, just learning how to perform free-weight exercises properly can lead to big increases in strength, says Armstrong Atlantic State University's Dr. Bob Lefavi.

"This stems from what we call the neuromuscular learning that occurs in the first three to five weeks of training," Dr. Lefavi says. "Just learning how to do a squat or press a bar in a bench press straight up in a biomechanically efficient pattern takes skill, forces your muscles to adapt, and results in increased force production."

The Overload Principle

Okay, so you've found a gym with iron to spare—and preferably one that has the owner's name in the title. (Our personal, all-time favorite: Johnny Lats.) Now what? It would probably be a good idea to plan your exercise routine. And especially if you want to slash time from your workout, forget the movements that only isolate small muscles that you can't even pronounce. Stick with basic movements that exercise several big muscles at a time: squats, leg presses, lunges, bench presses, military presses, seated rows or lat pull-downs, and, if you have the time, a set of curls, tricep extensions, and abdominal curls.

"If your training time is really limited, there's no question that doing a leg press rather than knee extensions and knee curls is the way to go. You cover all those bases with one exercise," says Dr. Fleck. And those exercises aren't better just because they more closely mimic the movements that you might do on the softball diamond or during a soccer game.

"If you think about it, you're doing more work per rep, so you're going to get more out of it in terms of changing your body composition," says Michael Stone, Ph.D., professor of exercise science at Appalachian State University in Boone, North Carolina, and president of the National Strength and Conditioning Association.

Perhaps the most important principle to remember when training for strength is that you

Benching the Bench Press

The University of Nebraska football team is known for brute strength, not finesse. And one of the most time-honored measures of brute strength is the bench press. Talk about a hot prospect, and usually the first things you hear are his maximum bench press and his 40-yard sprint time. But not in the Cornhuskers weight room.

That's because the players are too busy pumping iron on the Hammer Jammer, one of several revolutionary exercise machines developed by equipment manufacturer Hammer Strength in conjunction with Nebraska's football program.

"I'm not big on machines, but this is probably going to catch on like wildfire, because it's based on biomechanics—the way the body works," says the University of Nebraska's Boyd Epley.

Unlike traditional exercise machines, which usually feature a comfy seat and exercise only one muscle at a

need to lift heavy weights for a small number of repetitions. And by heavy, we mean a weight that's heavy to you—not what some gym rat has taken years to learn how to hoist. As a general rule of thumb, if you can lift the weight for more than six reps, it's not heavy enough for strength training.

And if you're a beginner, you don't have to knock yourself out with a million sets either. In fact, for folks who have just started working out, at least one study shows that performing one set is nearly as good as doing three to increase strength.

Researchers at the University of Florida in Gainesville had 38 folks who had never worked out before do leg extensions three times a week for 14 weeks. All used as much weight as they could handle, but half did three sets, and the rest performed just one set. As it turned out, both groups experienced similar im-

time, the new equipment harnesses what Epley calls ground-based technology—in other words, the seats have been removed, and you're forced to stand on your own two feet while performing the exercise.

As a result, the new machines force you to train several muscles at once in movements that are similar to those you make on the gridiron. "For the Hammer Jammer, think of a bench, but instead of lying flat, you're vertical, feet on the ground and body erect, and there's no back to it," Epley says. "You develop your strength by stabilizing your body and forcing your arms forward—just as you would out on the football field. And let me tell you, if you can develop that force, now you have something that's going to help win football games."

And that good old-fashioned gauge of manly strength, the bench press? "We don't even recognize that lift as one of the important ones anymore," Epley says.

your way up again," he says.

A common mistake among both beginners and more advanced trainers in their quest for brute strength is trying to train with heavy weights every workout. Instead, you'll want to alternate heavy and light workouts during the week. For example, if you did heavy bench presses on Monday, you'll want to go light on Wednesday so that your muscles can recover and then, if you feel like you're ready, go heavy again on Friday.

Another common problem is adding *too* much weight. "You're curling 40 pounds and then decide to go up 10 pounds, but that's a 25 percent increase—a huge jump, especially for curls," says Dr. Fleck.

Instead, add no more than 5 to 10 percent of the weight you're already using and don't go up again until you're lifting that weight for six reps. Just recognize that as the months pass, it's likely that your gains will plateau.

"As you get in better shape, the gains are going to get smaller, and it might be every two weeks before you're able to add some weight. Getting stronger becomes a harder task," Dr. Fleck cautions.

Depending on how much you've worked out in the past, you may find that you've reached your strength plateau between 6 and 12 weeks after you've started. Don't worry. More gains lie ahead, as long as you're willing to change your routine. Now may be the perfect time to switch to a higher-rep, lighter-weight routine designed to help build muscle.

One classic strength-building cycle performed at the University of Nebraska goes like this: "You build a base with somewhat higher reps (8 to 12) for three or four weeks, then you focus on strength for three or four weeks, and then you want to peak for two or three weeks. That's going to improve your performance no matter what sport you're in," says Epley.

provements in strength and size—but the single-set group was hitting the showers a lot quicker than the other.

Whether you do one set or three, you still have to continue to overload your muscles if you want to gain strength. "No question about it, if you want growth in strength, there has to be overload," Epley says. "And once again, most fitness programs don't do that."

But how much overload do you need? More good news for the time-pressed: not a heck of a lot. "Let's say that you're able to do three sets of six reps of a bench press with 185 pounds, your body weight," says Dr. Fleck. "If you wanted to get stronger, you'd add 10 pounds the next week and do as many as you could. Chances are that you'd be able to do three or four reps. But you'd stay at that weight until you could do three sets of six reps again. Then you'd add 10 pounds more and work

An Aerobic Exercise Primer

Feel the Burn— And the Afterburn

When you last rejected aerobics as an exercise option, there were probably enough good reasons to create your own Top Ten List.

10. Tired of taking orders from women
9. Richard Simmons
8. Cigar smoking frowned upon
7. Fat people in spandex make you squeamish
6. Compared to you, Al Gore looks as graceful on the dance floor as Fred Astaire
5. Find thong outer garments constricting
4. Risk almost certain expulsion from bowling team
3. Not enough room on bench step for beer stein
2. No halftime
1. Susan Powter

All reasonable, rational considerations, to be sure. But aerobic exercise is a lot more than stepping in time like an extra in a Michael Jackson video. In fact, even walking briskly around the block, swatting tennis balls, swimming at a moderate pace, and weekend chores like raking leaves or cutting the grass with a power push mower (*not* your John Deere riding tractor) qualify.

Of course, with an aerobic exercise routine like that, it's unlikely that anyone will ever mistake you for a triathlete. The point is that aerobic exercise doesn't mean squeezing into spandex and

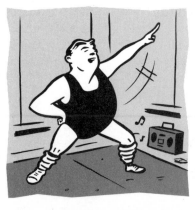

sweating to the oldies. It's any exercise that works your heart and lungs, or cardiorespiratory system.

The basic concept behind building cardiorespiratory fitness is essentially the same as for building muscle. You work the heart, forcing it to pump blood more efficiently, and the lungs, increasing their ability to provide oxygen. And the health benefits cannot be overstated. Even moderate activity such as walking has been found to help prevent health problems like heart disease, diabetes, and high blood pressure.

The Next Level

Significantly improving your cardiorespiratory fitness with aerobic exercise is another matter. Experts say that it takes raising your heart rate more often and to higher levels—between 60 and 90 percent of its maximum for anywhere from 20 to 60 minutes three or more times a week—to really see the fitness benefits of aerobic conditioning.

But here's where the cross-training revolution comes in. Many activities—from boxing and bicycling to treadmill walking—performed with the right intensity, can get you there.

"Really the most important thing is just to find some kind of aerobic exercise that you enjoy participating in. They all pretty much provide the same benefits if the appropriate intensity is reached," says Laura Gladwin of Brea, California, director of certification and training for the American Fitness Association, the world's largest fitness education organization.

What's more, aerobic exercise gives you the option of working out alone without any equipment—like a solitary, after-hours jog through a deserted downtown. Or popping a workout video into your VCR in the comfort and privacy of your home (safe from the disapproving glare of your bowling pals) when you don't have time to get to the gym.

And if you don't mind spending a few bucks to lift your aerobic exercise program to a new level of sophistication, you can incorporate a heart rate monitor into your routine.

"Heart rate monitors are changing the whole face of aerobic exercise as we know it, because they can make people successful at any level," says Amy Nelson, president of Heart Aerobics and a certified health/fitness instructor based in Los Angeles who has helped choreograph exercise videos featuring Kathy Smith and the National Aerobics Champions.

The New Face of Aerobics

It launched a fitness revolution in the early 1980s, sending women scurrying to newly sprouted fitness studios like so many spandex-clad Stepford wives. In response, most men yawned, scratched themselves, and went back to another recent invention, ESPN.

But since then, aerobics has morphed into a fat-burning, power-building workout that's among the best at increasing cardiorespiratory fitness. A little rhythm still helps, and there are still plenty of pretty women bouncing around, but it's fair to say that this ain't just a fancy dance class anymore. "It's been a gradual evolution from the early choreography to more advanced stuff and now plyometric and strength conditioning," Nelson says.

A plyometric bench-step workout, for example, has you jumping onto a bench "like a vertical jump you would use playing basketball," says Nelson. "Track athletes do this when they train. And you always jump up, never down, to avoid undue impact forces to your joints."

The increasing use of heart rate monitors

Heavenly Advice

You've died and gone to workout heaven: All the exercise machines at your gym are available. Which piece do you pick if you want the best workout?

If you want to burn calories, you can't go wrong with the treadmill, a clear winner by far in a joint study conducted by researchers at the Medical College of Wisconsin and the Clement J. Zablocki Veterans Affairs Medical Center, both in Milwaukee. But if you're looking for cardiovascular benefit, you might want to consider the VersaClimber, a machine similar to a stairclimber that works the upper body at the same time.

In the first study, treadmill users walking or "running somewhat hard" burned 705 calories an hour; those on a stair-climbing machine burned 627, and those using a rower burned 606. The next most efficient was the cross-country ski machine, with 595 calories spent in an hour. Those who used a bike machine that works both arms and legs burned 509 calories, while the stationary bike ranked dead last, with just 498 calories burned in an hour.

But when researchers at Washington State University in Seattle compared the results of athletes who trained on a treadmill, a rowing machine, and a VersaClimber, those who trained on the VersaClimber had higher heart rates and used more oxygen.

is helping overcome the rap against group aerobics that there was no way to know whether you had pushed yourself to a new level of fitness.

"A heart rate monitor gives you a window on your insides in a noninvasive way, without taking blood lactates, a urinalysis, or a muscle biopsy. You can see how hard you're working, and then you can tailor your exercise toward your goals," says Nelson.

As a result, a growing number of aerobic exercisers alternate hard, easy, and moderate training days, just like their body-building and strength-training brethren. "We want to get fitter and better, but we go out and do the same things day after day and wonder why we don't get results," Nelson says. "But if you're designing a training program, you should look at the week and say, 'This is my total time. How should I vary my intensity level throughout the week?' "

The Great Aerobic Exercise Divide

According to a preliminary study, just how you divide your aerobic exercise time can result in radically different results. Researchers at San Jacinto College in Houston found that of 67 people who performed aerobics for 15 weeks, those who worked out twice a week for 60 minutes had greater cardiovascular gains than people who worked out three times a week for 40 minutes. That's one less workout a week—a veritable vacation for someone pressed for time.

If trimming inches and pounds are your goal, however, you may want to stick with the three-days-a-week plan. The folks on that schedule lost 3.7 inches from their thighs, biceps, waist, and chest. People working out twice a week lost less than half an inch over the same time period.

"It makes sense," says Michael Soileau, Ed.D., a health and physical education expert at San Jacinto College in Houston and author of the study. "Let's say that you're going to work out an hour a week. If you were to break that workout up into six 10-minute workouts, you would burn more calories than you would if you worked out for one 60-minute workout, simply because your body burns more calories after you exercise. We call that afterburn of calories. So in our study, the group that lost the most got three afterburns instead of two."

To get another picture of how powerful

On Target

Thanks to the miracle of modern technology, there are now two ways to check your heart rate. The old low-tech way is as simple as holding your finger on your neck or the underside of your wrist until you can feel a pulse, counting the beats for 10 seconds and multiplying by 6.

Fortunately for those of us with fleshy necks and wrists and limited math skills, several companies manufacture wireless heart rate monitors. Featuring a transmitter belt that's worn around the chest and a wristwatchlike receiver that displays a digital readout, wireless heart monitors literally give a second-by-second account of your heart rate.

And when used properly, the information is invaluable. "It's techno-training—the difference between the telegraph and e-mail," says Amy Nelson of Heart Aerobics. "We used to say, 'Let's stop, take our heart rate . . . oh, I missed it. Oh, I can't feel my pulse.' You want to know how hard you're working, but when you have to stop for 10

the afterburn effect can be, consider this University of Missouri study. Researchers discovered that seven active men who bicycled for an hour burned 600 calories during a workout and 120 extra calories in the nine hours following the workout.

If only aerobic exercise worked as well at helping to build muscle and strength. "There is this underlying philosophy that you get some kind of muscle strength and power component to standard bench stepping, for example," says Thomas E. Dohmeier, Ph.D., director of research at Condell Medical Health Center Institute in Libertyville, Illinois. "Guys who do a lot of aerobic activity are going to lose some body fat, and they are going to lose some weight. But the only way that you're going to increase your strength doing this type of activity is to increase the weight somehow. Plyometrics builds power, and there's a difference."

seconds to find out, it's counterproductive."

But if strapping on a heart rate monitor is easy, figuring out your maximum heart rate and, as a result, your target heart rate is a little more difficult.

"The short answer for max heart rate is 220 minus your age, but that's only right about 50 percent of the time," says Nelson, who also travels the country giving seminars on how to determine an accurate heart rate.

For maximum fat burning and cardiorespiratory benefit, it's important to keep your heart rate between 60 and 90 percent of its maximum for anywhere from 20 to 60 minutes three or more times a week. To estimate your minimum target heart rate, subtract your age from 220 and then multiply by 0.60. To estimate your maximum target heart rate, subtract your age from 220 and then multiply by 0.90. Just remember that this estimate has been found to vary by 15 to 20 beats per minute.

Unfortunately, holding hand weights while you jog or do aerobics doesn't cut it. Squeezing the weight acts as a tourniquet, compressing your arteries, slowing blood flow, and, as a result, taking your heart out of its training zone, says Mark L. Bailey, Ph.D., an exercise physiologist in the Human Performance Lab in the Department of Physical Education at California State University, Los Angeles.

Riding the Circuit

If you still wouldn't be caught dead in an aerobics class and don't have time for separate strength training and aerobic workouts, you may want to consider circuit training.

With some of the cardiovascular benefits of an aerobics class and the potential for strength gain and muscle toning besides, circuit training is one of the most popular programs used by personal trainers to get busy clients in shape.

"Circuit training is the preferred method of training for people who are busy because you can combine cardiovascular training with strength training and still keep your heart rate in your target zone," says Bill Kyser, a spokesman for the Fitness Products Council and a personal trainer based in Boca Raton, Florida.

A typical circuit training session includes 12 to 20 exercises performed at 40 to 50 percent of your one-rep maximum for 30 seconds. Like a product on an assembly line, you proceed to the next workout station, rest for 30 seconds, and then exercise for another 30 seconds. The circuit is repeated two to four times, depending on the individual's fitness level.

But just like more intense aerobic workouts, the goal is to keep your heart rate within the fat-burning, heart-building target zone of 60 to 90 percent of its maximum for the entire workout.

According to Kyser, a beginner's circuit-training workout doesn't have to last more than 20 minutes, while an intermediate or more advanced athlete can make solid strength gains with an hour of circuit training. In fact, one Navy study showed that men who performed a 10-week circuit-training program improved the muscular endurance of their bench press—the number of times they could lift 60 percent of their one-rep max—by nearly 40 percent, while their work capacity on a stationary bike improved by 3 percent.

As that study indicates, circuit training can provide a slight boost to cardiovascular fitness, but it's no substitute for aerobic work.

"Circuit training in theory is good, but it just isn't as good as pure cardiovascular exercise," says Larry Gibbons, M.D., president of the Cooper Institute for Aerobics Research in Dallas.

A Stretching Primer

How to Be a Flexible Guy

It's not going to put Pike-size peaks on your biceps, boost your endurance, or otherwise whip you into fighting trim. There's even some argument about whether stretching—even as part of an athletic training program—improves performance.

But if you'd like to keep your body flexible, you can't beat stretching. And, perhaps more important, if you haven't found the time to work out for a while, some experts suggest that a quick stretching break may help lure you back to the gym.

"People with sedentary jobs sometimes have trouble bridging the gap between their work—which really makes them tired—and then going for a run, workout, or bike ride. They just don't want to do anything," says Bob Anderson, stretching expert, author of *Stretching at Your Computer or Desk* and *Stretching*, and co-author of *Getting in Shape*. "A few gentle stretches make you feel better and put you in touch with your body. And if that doesn't make you want to work out, I don't know what will," says Anderson.

Although it's a proven tension reliever and muscle relaxer, lots of guys go out of their way to avoid stretching. "Unless they're really flexible, most guys aren't into it," Anderson says. "And because women tend to be a lot more flexible than men, they don't like to stretch around them much."

But if you're concerned that you'll have to assume lotus-like positions or otherwise con-

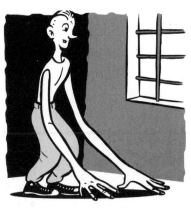

tort yourself to produce the best stretching results, Anderson says to relax. "It's not like you have to be able to put your foot behind your head or do splits. You should simply try to incorporate stretching into your life and then free yourself up from having to always do more, to stretch farther every time. The most important thing is to stretch those tissues correctly," says Anderson.

The Right Stretch

Like to gnaw on the end of a chicken drumstick? That rubbery stuff on the end is the cartilage that makes up the joint—virtually the same as what you have at the ends of your bones. In a healthy joint, a thin lining called the synovium releases a lubricating fluid that works better than WD-40 at keeping it loose and mobile. But the less you move, the less lubrication is released. After years of inactivity—like parking yourself in front of a computer or TV screen—your joints can stiffen or even freeze when muscles and tendons become too weak or too tight to allow movement.

Any careful exercise—be it riding a mountain bike, pumping some iron, or taking a nice long hike—will obviously help lubricate your joints and keep them healthy. But what if you've been chained to a desk for the last two decades? You may be able to regain some of the lost flexibility by stretching.

Unlike most athletic pursuits, which continuously stress ever-greater achievement like running faster, lifting more, or throwing farther, stretching in its purest form simply requires your most comfortable effort.

"A lot of people say, 'I'm going to do my stretching exercises.' But as soon as you put exercise with the word *stretch*, you miss the whole point," Anderson says. "Some people can touch their toes, and others can't go beyond their knees. I say that both people are doing it right. One of the last things you want to do is compare flexibility with someone else."

But there are proper ways to perform the movements. Whenever you stretch, push yourself only until you feel mild tension. Without bouncing, hold the stretch for 5 to 15 seconds. Try to breathe slowly and naturally. "The tension should ease as you hold the stretch," Anderson says.

For increased flexibility, "stretch a fraction of an inch farther until you feel mild tension, and hold it for 5 to 15 seconds," says Anderson. Once again, don't bounce. And don't stretch too far. "Stretching muscle fibers too far causes a nerve reflex to signal for the muscle to contract," Anderson says.

Instead of randomly stretching a few body parts and then moving to your chosen activity, take a few minutes to stretch complementary muscle areas. "All the upper-body stretches should be done at the same time. Or all the sitting stretches. They should all kind of flow one from another. I think it's easier to remember them that way," Anderson says.

And here's a valuable time-saving tip for weight training. You can use the time between sets to lightly stretch the muscle you've just trained. "Not really hard and heavy stretches that push you as far as you can go. Just lightly stretch the muscles that you have just used for 8 to 10 seconds. And then go back and use them again. I think what it does is keep the range that you started with," Anderson says.

The jury is still out on whether stretching a cold muscle can cause injury, but Anderson believes that it's safe. "As long as you know how to stretch your own body and you go by the feeling of the stretch—the one that says, 'I'm comfortable, I'm in control'—you should be

Stretching the Workday

Working on the railroad all the live-long day used to be tough on the back and shoulders of Burlington Northern Santa Fe conductor Gary Jerman.

His company's solution: stretching. All 44,000 employees are not only required to perform stretches during their workday but also are taught proper technique.

"Let's say that you've been riding the train and sitting for two hours. You're supposed to stretch before you perform your next task," says Jerman, of Sterling, Colorado. "We're supposed to perform them before every shift, before any task, and after any relaxed time, so to speak."

Designed by the company's in-house medical department in conjunction with stretching expert Bob Anderson, the program has helped keep Jerman—a recreational runner who logs between 12 and 15 miles a week—injury-free. But according to him, that may not even be the best part.

"You know what else is neat? Anytime I go to a big safety meeting where there are big company officials, we all do our stretching. Before the meeting and after we come back from lunch. They're that serious about it," Jerman says.

okay," Anderson says. "I'm not saying don't warm up. I'm saying that if you know what you're doing, you don't need any elaborate warm-up."

For those who intend to try to increase their flexibility with more rigorous stretching, always warm up, Anderson says. Riding a bike or jogging slowly for five minutes or until you break a sweat should be enough, he says. "If you're going to work on this hyperflexibility stuff, you don't have an option. Warm up first."

Putting the Pieces Together

How to Set—And Achieve—Your Goals

When management consultant Dr. Kenneth Blanchard, author of the business classic *The One-Minute Manager*, first observed that no one on their deathbed ever wished they had spent more time at the office, he was challenging us to strike the right balance between our work and personal lives.

"We let our lives be run by the urgent—our voice mail, our e-mail, that kind of thing," Dr. Blanchard says. "The key is bumping your health up so that it's not just important; it's urgent like faith and family. And keeping it there."

But once you've determined that your health and fitness is a priority, you have another challenge. In the myriad of exercise options—like running and stretching and swimming and weight training—how do you strike the right balance?

The Basics

In large measure, that decision is probably determined by your fitness goals—what you plan to accomplish with your limited exercise time. For the less ambitious, that may mean trying to get by with the bare minimum needed to avoid health problems. For others, we could be talking about an exercise program that stretches and challenges you more as the years go by.

First, though, it's probably a good idea to make sure that you have certain basic health bases covered.

If you smoke, quit. It's true that smokers who are aerobically fit actually live longer than otherwise healthy sofa spuds who don't smoke. But that probably has more to do with the power of exercise than the documented dangers of smoking. Whether it's dramatically reducing your risk for deadly disease such as lung cancer or emphysema or improving your cardiovascular function—strengthening your heart and lungs—kicking those butts does it all.

"And if you can't stop cold turkey, at least start to cut back. If you're smoking two packs, smoke one pack. If you're smoking one pack, smoke half a pack," says Charles Kuntzleman, Ed.D., professor of kinesiology at the University of Michigan in Ann Arbor and director of Blue Cross and Blue Shield of Michigan Fitness for Youth Program, also at the University of Michigan.

Move it or lose it. So, once and for all, how much exercise do you need to improve your health? Thirty minutes—roughly one insipid prime-time sitcom and several annoying commercials—three or more times a week.

"It could be three 10-minute bouts; it could be two 15-minute bouts; it could be six 5-minute bouts," says Dr. Kuntzleman. "And you should really think that way. If you haven't done anything, you need to say, 'Okay, the key element here is for me to get 30 minutes of moderate exercise today somehow. That's the bottom line.' "

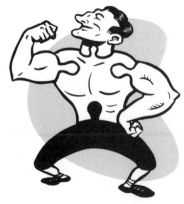

And while one man's definition of moderate exercise may be the dash between the fridge and the couch, the actual recommendation is walking at a pace that's about 3.5 miles per hour.

Practice moderation. Some studies show a link between moderate drinking—one to two drinks a day—and reduced risk for heart disease. But there's absolutely no suggestion that even more would be better. "And if you're a teetotaler or drink less than that, you shouldn't suddenly start drinking. What they're saying is that if you're drinking less than that, stay there. But if you're consuming more than that, you should cut back," Dr. Kuntzleman says.

Getting Ready to Run

Let's assume for a moment that you've taken the first steps: You don't smoke, you're exercising three to five days a week, and you're having no more than two drinks a day.

Even though you may be feeling fitter than ever, if you've been recliner-bound for several years, you probably shouldn't add much more exercise to your fitness program for the next 12 weeks.

"It's like the guy who used one bag of fertilizer on his lawn and it looked great, so he used another bag and it killed the grass," says Dr. Kuntzleman. "That's the problem with fitness for people who haven't been active. They think, 'This makes me feel so good, now I'm really going to get after it.' And they end up with all kinds of orthopedic problems, knee problems, and hip problems. It may not occur right away but a year or two later when their body finally breaks down."

Once you've built that 12-week base, however, then it's probably time to branch out. If you've been walking regularly, you could start by combining walking and running—five minutes of running if you're over 40, 10 minutes if you are under 40, says Dr. Kuntzleman. Then increase the amount of time that you're running by one minute a week.

Running a 10-K

While dutifully doing your roadwork on your treadmill at the gym one day, you notice an application for a local 10-K road race. A debate rages in your head. Could I make it? Would it be fun? Will I really get a free T-shirt?

Believe it or not, with several months of

walking and running under your training belt, you're only about four weeks of training away from crossing the finish line—and proudly claiming your free T-shirt. Simply increase your running to five days a week and follow this schedule recommended by Armstrong Atlantic State University's Dr. Bob Lefavi.

Week One

Sunday: Run for 30 to 45 minutes at an easy pace that's slow enough so that you can carry on a conversation with a partner.

Monday: Rest.

Tuesday: Run easily for 10 minutes to warm up. Next, quicken your pace for 5 minutes, then jog for 5 minutes, speed up for another 5, then slow down a bit for 5 minutes. Cool down with 10 minutes of easy jogging.

Wednesday and Thursday: Run easily for 15 to 30 minutes.

Friday: Take a 10-minute warm-up jog. Then run up a 100- to 200-yard hill at a modest pace five times and at your race pace five times, recovering with a slow jog on the way down. Finish with a 10-minute cooldown.

Saturday: Rest.

Weeks Two and Three

Repeat the week one workout, but increase your Sunday runs by 15 minutes each week, picking up your pace slightly.

Week Four (Race Week)

Sunday: Run for 45 to 60 minutes at an easy pace.

Monday: Rest.

Tuesday: Warm up for 10 minutes. Alternate 2 minutes of race-pace running with 3 minutes of easy jogging for three cycles. Cool down for 10 minutes.

Wednesday: Rest.

Thursday and Friday: Do 15 to 30 minutes of easy running.

Saturday: Rest or jog easily for 10 minutes to keep your legs loose.

Sunday: Race. Have fun. And don't forget to pick up your T-shirt.

Here are some quick tips on racing smart. Above all, don't start too fast. The idea is to cover the distance, not finish in the top 10. If you're gasping for breath, it's okay to walk for a while; many runners do in a race this long. You can always pick up the pace as you approach the finish. Okay, so you have 200 yards left to go and you're feeling strong. Start your kick. To squeeze more speed from your body, try this trick. Pick a runner 20 yards in front of you and hunt him down like a greyhound after a rabbit. Blow past him at the finish line. Once you cross, grab a cup of water and walk for 5 to 10 minutes.

Swim a Mile

Assuming you haven't forgotten how to swim, this program will turn you into a tuna in 30 days.

Find a 25-yard lap pool, swim one length, and count your strokes. "If you take more than 20 arm strokes, you should improve your stroke efficiency first," says Terry Laughlin, director of the Total Immersion national swimming camps for adults, based in Goshen, New York. "For novices, swimming is at least 80 percent proper mechanics. It's not swimming faster; it's swimming easier."

The keys are lengthening your stroke and keeping your hips and legs from dragging. "Try leaning your chest more so that it feels as if you are swimming downhill," Laughlin says. "That'll keep your hips and legs near the surface so that you'll be more streamlined."

Here are two tricks for lengthening your stroke. As each arm enters the water, reach—just as you would for something on a high shelf—before starting your pull. And roll your hips from side to side with each stroke. "Your hips, not your shoulders, are your engines," Laughlin says.

Here's the workout. Swim one or two

The Ride of a Century

Every September, cyclists take to the streets to perform organized 100-mile rides to celebrate National Century Month. And with a little effort, you could be one of them.

Of course, riding 100 miles is probably a tall order for anyone to prepare for in a month—even a guy with a solid fitness base like you. So why not try a shorter trek? One of the most popular for beginning cyclists is the 100-kilometer (62-mile) metric century. To find a century ride near you, inquire at your local bike shop.

The following training schedule was recommended by Armstrong Atlantic State University's Dr. Bob Lefavi. It's a proven program that has helped thousands of cyclists just

	Mon. (Easy)	Tues. (Pace)	Wed. (Brisk)
Week One	6	10	12
Week Two	7	11	13
Week Three	8	13	15
Week Four	8	14	17
Week Five	8	14	17

lengths, practicing the moves mentioned above, then rest. Repeat this routine for 30 to 40 minutes three times a week. When you can swim 100 yards in 80 strokes or less, you can start building sets of 100-yard repeats, resting for 15 to 30 seconds between 100-yard swims. Once you can swim about 18 of these, you're ready to attempt a mile swim. That's 1,760 yards, or about 71 laps in a 25-yard pool. To beat the boredom of lap swimming, swim your mile in a lake, with a buddy rowing a boat ahead of you for safety.

Flex Appeal

You've never been much of a team player, and you get no kick out of running or

like you meet the challenge.

Note: "Easy" means a leisurely ride. "Pace" means matching the speed you hope to maintain during the metric century. (Depending on how hilly the course is, you can expect a 62-mile century ride to take you between four and six hours, so plan your pace accordingly.) "Brisk" means riding at least 2 miles per hour faster than your century speed.

It's important to ride at least five days per week. If you skip a day, make sure that it's not a Saturday, your long-mileage day. Covering greater distances each weekend is key. If weather or something else derails your Saturday ride, use Sunday as the long day.

Thurs.	Fri. (Pace)	Sat. (Pace)	Sun. (Pace)	Weekly Mileage
Off	10	30	9	77
Off	11	34	10	86
Off	13	38	11	98
Off	14	42	13	108
Off	10	5 (easy)	Century Race	116

riding a bike. But you've always been a stickler for details, and now that you're lifting weights, you love to feel the burn. Bodybuilding could be for you.

"Maybe the best way to describe it is that a bodybuilder needs to look at his body as a sculpture," says Dr. Lefavi. "You need to be able to look at yourself and say, 'I need more work here or a little less there,' and then train with that in mind."

Of course, you also have to start with the basics. Here's how it's done when you don't have all day.

Train to fatigue. For one to three sets per exercise, train with a weight that makes you quit somewhere between 8 and 12 reps. "If you can't reach 8, the weight is probably too heavy;

if you do more than 12 easily, your weight is too light," says Dr. Lefavi.

Give yourself a day off. After a workout, your muscles need about 48 to 72 hours to rebuild and recover, says Dr. Lefavi. That means, at least at first, you shouldn't work out with weights more than three times a week. In fact, it's best to weight-train two or three times a week on nonconsecutive days, he says.

Try something new. When Dr. Lefavi coaches beginning and even seasoned bodybuilders, he challenges them to ask this question before they walk into the gym: What can I do differently this time?

"If you don't have adequate, intense stimulation of your muscles, there is no growth," Dr. Lefavi says. "So that means you should constantly do things differently—trying new exercises, for example. Or even doing the same routine in different order. Instead of chest first, do legs. Instead of back first, biceps. That provides the body with what we call an adequate alarm to help promote growth."

Plan ahead. After training like this for three to four months, you've laid a solid foundation. But if you're thinking about participating in a local bodybuilding contest, it's probably best to find one that's nine months to a year away.

"When I was competing, I looked a year ahead and mapped out where I wanted to be by then in terms of body weight, strength, percentage of body fat, posing ability, and how I could tailor my routines and diet to meet those goals," Dr. Lefavi says. "But I would also set specific milestones along the way that helped to motivate me and were achievable. This keeps you focused and gives you the opportunity to go back in time and look at a record and plan and look at what routines you were doing at the time when you had the greatest growth."

Signing Up for Health Benefits

Exercise Is Key for a Longer, Better Life

We're a nation of multi-taskers. Scanning magazines while we eat. Chatting on cellular phones while we commute. Reading the newspaper while we watch TV. And just wait until some genius opens a chain of drive-thru fast-food joints that will dry-clean your suit, quick-lube your car, and offer you instant cash from an automated teller machine—all in the time it takes to bag your burger and fries.

Yet many of us ignore the ultimate time-saver: fitness. Unlike shortcuts that trim mere seconds or minutes from our crazed schedules, regular exercise does something far better: It actually *adds* quality and years to your life.

How much? If a 30-year-old, two-packs-a-day smoker with high cholesterol kicked the smoking habit, changed his diet, and started exercising regularly, he'd add 8 to 10 years to his life, says Kenneth G. Manton, Ph.D., research professor and director of Duke University's Center for Demographic Studies in Durham, North Carolina.

How's that for time management? There's not a thing you can do that will add even one second to your day. At the end of 24 hours, it's over. But exercise and good nutrition can literally add years to your life.

"Regular exercise is positively linked to so many things," says Dr. Manton. "It can affect blood pressure. It affects caloric balance and body

mass, total cholesterol levels . . . you name it."

And when it comes to reducing stress, boosting energy levels, even improving your attitude, fitness has few equals.

"Ten years ago we thought that exercise was important," explains Dr. Larry Gibbons of the Cooper Institute for Aerobics Research. "Today the evidence is so solid that anybody who wants to enjoy good health has to be exercising regularly. It's no longer an option. It is essential."

Fit for Life

If you're still inclined to spend your spare time in a recliner, consider the alternative. As many as 250,000 deaths each year—about 12 percent of total deaths—are attributable, in part, to a lack of regular physical activity. As a risk factor, experts say that physical inactivity is just as bad as smoking, hypertension, and high cholesterol.

But research shows that you don't have to spend your life in a gym to take advantage of the benefits of exercise. In the landmark Harvard alumni study, researchers found that death rates declined as the number of calories burned per week rose from 500 to 3,500. Death rates were a third lower among those alumni who burned more than 2,000 calories a week exercising—roughly the equivalent of walking three miles a day.

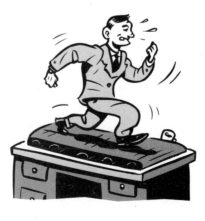

"We know from both short-term and long-term studies that you really get a lot of health benefits from being active, even at the level of brisk walking," says Michael Pratt, M.D., acting chief for the physical activity and health branch in the National Center for Chronic Disease Prevention and Health Promotion of the Centers for Disease Control and Prevention in Atlanta. "And in virtually all those studies we're finding that the biggest benefit is for those who go from no exercise to some."

The Heart of the Matter

Some of the most convincing reasons to make sure that you cram a workout into your workday start with your heart. A study by the Cooper Institute in Dallas found that men who became fit over five years were 44 percent less likely to die from cardiovascular disease than those who didn't. "As it turned out, it was just as important for the men in this study to become fit as it was for them to stop smoking in order to protect against death," Dr. Gibbons says.

The Cooper Institute's definition of *fit* is simply pulling on a pair of walking shoes and hitting the bricks for an average of 30 minutes a day, three to five days a week. "Obviously, this is a level of fitness that's doable by virtually everyone. And, in fact, it's a very significant benefit even for those age 60 and above," Dr. Gibbons says.

Consider a study performed during the 1985 World Masters Games in Toronto. Researchers found that participants who took a cycling test—some of them 60 to 70 years old—had the cardiopulmonary fitness of sedentary 25-year-olds. And many of them trained less than seven hours a week. Other studies show that maximal performance of active folks remains unchanged for 20, 30, even 40 years—obviously a great way to stop the big hands on the aging clock.

Disease-Free

That's not all the bang you get for your exercise buck. Research also shows that colon

---

High-Five Your Anxiety

Got a deadline looming? Hitting the weights and the stair-climber won't keep your boss at bay, but research shows that it will probably help you manage your job stress better.

In one study conducted at California State University, Long Beach, researchers reported that volunteers who walked for just 10 minutes every morning for six days were more optimistic, happier, and felt better than those who walked in the late afternoon.

In another study, University of Chicago at Urbana-Champaign researchers found that volunteers who exercised more often—three or more times a week—were more optimistic and less anxious than those who rarely darkened a gym door. And in a victory for cross-training, those who both performed aerobic exercise and lifted weights reported even less anxiety than those strictly pumping iron.

---

cancer and diabetes rates plunge when folks find time for fitness. "Again, the reduction of risk is substantial: 30 to 100 percent reduction for both. Almost the same as for coronary heart disease," says Dr. Pratt.

In addition, when folks who had high blood pressure, which is a risk for both stroke and coronary heart disease, exercised on stationary bikes for 16 weeks, three times per week, for 30 to 60 minutes per exercise session at 60 to 80 percent of their maximum heart rate, both their systolic and diastolic blood pressure dropped substantially. These folks were even able to reduce their blood pressure medication by 40 percent.

And although men are clearly at less risk for osteoporosis than women, weight training throughout your life virtually eliminates the chance by boosting bone density.

Fitness and Sex

Making the Love Connection

Sorry, pal. Even at its panting, rip-each-other's-clothes-off best, sex isn't much of a workout.

In fact, research shows that the average 15-minute interlude is comparable to trudging up two flights of stairs—a trip that probably burns less than 60 calories. With paltry numbers like that, you'd have to rise to the occasion four times just to burn off a cup of low-fat strawberry yogurt. And that Snickers bar you just devoured? Don't ask.

"The reality is that it's nearly impossible when you're having sex to reach the physiological threshold of evoking cardiovascular benefit," says Tommy Boone, Ph.D., chairman of the Department of Exercise Physiology and director of the human performance laboratory at the College of St. Scholastica in Duluth, Minnesota.

In other words, sex may make your heart beat faster, but it won't help it beat longer. However, that's not to say that there's no connection between sex and fitness. Because one of the fastest ways to improve your sex life is regular exercise.

What Women Really Want

Make no mistake: Women above all want to be loved, honored, cherished, worshiped, and—to the extent that we guys are capable—understood.

But when they look under the hood, women are a lot like us: They like to see a beautiful bod. Or at least, that's the conclusion of a study of college women at Oregon State University in Corvallis. They ranked a man's build ahead of his eyes, face, height, and hair as the most im-portant characteristic of a good-looking guy. Their favorite body part: men's butts.

No surprise, this. But there may be a deeper reason than mere sexual attraction at play here, says Anthony Walsh, Ph.D., a psychobiologist at Boise State University in Idaho and author of the book *The Science of Love.* "A well-honed body is a clue to the health of the person owning it," Dr. Walsh says. "And certainly in terms of history, the fittest dude around probably controlled the most territory. And if you controlled the most territory, you could support the greatest number of offspring. And that's what females throughout the animal and human kingdom are looking for: provision of resources."

Why else, Dr. Walsh asks, would research show that newly minted female physicians want someone with even higher earning potential?

The bottom line is that you may not be able to rush out and earn a Ph.D. But after a few months of working out, you may just find yourself turning more heads.

Better in Bed

The next time you're thinking about skipping your workout because you're too busy, ask yourself this question: Are you too busy to have sex?

We can guess the answer. Well, Bubba, better hit the gym. Because there is growing research that shows a direct link between exercise and sex. And we're talking quantity *and* quality.

Researchers at the University of California, San Diego, randomly divided 95 middle-age men into two groups. Seventy-eight of the men biked, jogged, or used the trampoline at 75 to 80 percent of their maximum aerobic capacity an average of 60 minutes for 3.5 days a week. The rest walked in a group 60 minutes a day for 4.1 days a week.

Nine months later, the aerobic exercisers reported a 25 to 30 percent increase in their sexual activity across the board. Not only did these guys have sex more frequently, but they also had more orgasms per interlude, a higher percentage of satisfying orgasms, more desire for sex, and more reliable sexual function—and less body fat to boot. Meanwhile, the walkers averaged no real change in sexual activity or sexual function.

Researchers attribute the positive changes among the aerobics crew to a number of factors. "Improved blood flow and better oxygen delivery to the tissues is probably the most important factor for better erections," says David Case, Ph.D., associate research specialist in the Department of Psychology at the University of California, San Diego. "And it could be that since the men were feeling stronger and healthier, they were psychologically more interested in sex. With reduced body fat, the aerobic bodybuilders may have been more appealing sexually to their partners. Short-term exercise is also thought to increase testosterone levels—the male sex hormone. It could be any of these mechanisms, but I think that it's probably a combination."

The kicker is that most of the guys were 40-something middle-management types who had been told that they were taking part in a program to help reduce their heart disease risk. "This they did, but I'm sure that the sex results were a pleasant side effect," Dr. Case says.

A far less formal study of Master's class swimmers—both men and women in their forties and fifties—found that those who trained an average of an hour a day four or five days a week reported having sex seven times a month.

But remember: Too much of a good thing can be a bad thing. And in this case, we're talking about training. Overtraining has been found to reduce sexual interest in some

Is Sweat Sexy?

Unlike many animals, human sweat doesn't seem to have chemical components built in that are needed to attract the opposite sex, says George Preti, Ph.D., adjunct associate professor in the dermatology department at the University of Pennsylvania and a researcher at Monell Chemical Senses Center, both in Philadelphia.

It's another story if you're just trying to get your wife pregnant, Dr. Preti says. "There is something in the underarm components—what we call the male axillary components—that can influence the length and timing of her menstrual cycle," he says.

Researchers made the discovery after collecting male sweat, mixing it with ethanol, and—get this—"rubbing it under the noses of women who had a history of abnormal cycle length," says Dr. Preti. "We found that after about eight weeks of exposure, the women who were receiving the male extract had a more regular menstrual cycle length than women who had a history of abnormal cycle lengths and were only receiving a placebo."

athletes, particularly long-distance runners, says Jay S. Schinfeld, M.D., associate professor of obstetrics and gynecology at Jefferson Medical College of Thomas Jefferson University in Philadelphia and chief of reproductive endocrinology and infertility at Abington Memorial Hospital in Abington, Pennsylvania. "Testosterone levels drop. You start to feel less sexual and more fatigued. The sexual problems associated with overexercising are well-documented," he says.

Actual mileage may vary, but for some male runners it seems that testosterone levels start dropping when they run more than 45 to 60 miles a week. "We're *not* talking about 45 minutes of active exercise three or four times a week," says Dr. Schinfeld.

Being a Shrewd Time Manager

Invest Wisely and Reap the Rewards

Talk to the experts, and you're almost certain to hear them say that you'll never find time for fitness. You have to *make* time.

But that's not exactly true. There's not a thing you can do to add even one lousy second to the 86,400 seconds we're all allotted each day.

The issue really boils down to time management—using those 86,400 seconds wisely and efficiently enough each day so that you can spare at least 1,800 of them for exercise. It's a matter of setting priorities. One national survey of men in their thirties and forties found that 67 percent include being healthy and fit in their personal definition of *success*.

Now, take a look around you. Are two-thirds of the guys you see healthy and fit? Not unless you're standing on the starting line of the Boston Marathon.

Time Is on Your Side

Being in great shape is something that we'd love to do . . . if we had the time. Well, if it's time you want, step right up. We've combed the nooks and crannies of life, searching for those moments that so quickly seem to fade into oblivion and we found . . . a nickel and a half-roll of wintergreen breath mints. No—those were under the sofa cushion. Talking to the experts, folks who manage time for a living, we've uncovered hours of extra time that you can place at your disposal. Starting right

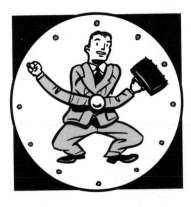

now. After all, there's no time like the present.

Get wise with your wardrobe. Maybe your mom made you lay out your clothes the night before school. Not a bad idea for big boys either, says Adele Pace, M.D., a fitness consultant in Ashland, Kentucky, and author of *The Busy Executive's Guide to Total Fitness.* For even faster dressing, you might want to consider organizing your closets and drawers, separating workout, work, and casual wear. If you're really a goof, consider the Jeff Goldblum approach. In the remake of the movie *The Fly*, Goldblum's mad-scientist character only owned identical jackets, pants, shirts, and shoes.

Put them back, Jack. According to one survey, office workers waste roughly 50 minutes a day searching for missing items. And truth be told, there's no way your home is as well-organized as your office. Instead of dropping things like your car keys, wallet, and sunglasses all over creation, find a regular place for them and then put them back after each use. You'll need those keys—and that time—to get to the gym.

Support free enterprise. While it's true that cutting the grass and raking leaves burn calories, if you're so pressed for time that you can't work out, you're almost better-off hiring the kid down the street to handle those chores. And not only will that help you find time for fitness but you'll also be teaching the lad the finer points of capitalism.

Appoint yourself promptly. Unless your barber took way too much off the top, there's no reason why you can't make another haircut appointment while you're there. Ditto for dentists or other services that require scheduling. It's either that or having to track down the phone number and make the call another time, which could eat into workout time on a particularly busy day.

Grow a beard. Okay, so it probably won't do much for your career—unless you plan to join ZZ Top or replace Jerry Garcia in the Grateful Dead. But surveys show that the average guy spends about 40 minutes a day grooming himself—at least 15 of which is spent shaving his face. And that's an extra 15 minutes you can use for increasing your cardio-vascular fitness. Not only that, but the money you save on shaving cream and razors can go for that pair of in-line skates you've always wanted.

Do your own delivery. The next time you find yourself waiting at Papa Luigi's for a large pizza to go, don't sit around watching the old man throw dough in the air. Take a walk. If you're extra ambitious, you may even want to consider—heaven forbid—walking up and back to the pizza shop. And make sure to ask for half the normal helping of cheese, unless you want to spend the next three workouts trying to burn it off.

Plan those holidays. Between shopping for gifts (a 6-hour affair) and the 10 hours on average spent arguing and bickering with family members about holiday-related activities, it's no wonder that you start to look like Santa. You can't find time to go to the gym. Rather than wandering through stores like an elf who's had too much egg nog, plan your Christmas purchases beforehand. And hey, here's a concept. Consider buying gifts the month *before* the big day.

Live by your list. The average grocery store visit takes 22 minutes. Can you do better? Maybe—if you make a list before you go and only shop in supermarkets that you know like the back of your hand. And no hanging around the bakery scrounging for free samples—it's bad for your abs.

Bring on breakfast. In a shortsighted attempt to get on the job early, many men skip breakfast and head straight for

In a Minute

With millions of copies in print, *The One-Minute Manager* is one of the world's best-selling management guides. Although management consultant and author Dr. Kenneth Blanchard wrote the book for corporate types, he says that most of his inquiries now come from those who are managing themselves.

"The business hierarchy is being broken down. People can't sit around and blame other folks for why things don't happen. They better take the initiative themselves. And I think that's always been true about health and exercise," Dr. Blanchard says.

Here are three keys that Dr. Blanchard says can help you save time and get in your workout.

One-minute goal setting. "All good perfor-mance—whether it's exercise or in the business world—starts with clear goals. Take a minute to figure out what you really want to do."

One-minute praising. "I've always felt that a lot of us don't praise ourselves enough. And sometimes you have to find yourself doing things approximately right. Not exactly right, but if you set a goal—like to make sure that you worked out or to run a certain distance—and you did it, pat yourself on the back."

One-minute reprimand. "When you don't do what you said you were going to do, you can reprimand your-self. Tell yourself how you feel about it. But then you have to always remember to reaffirm yourself. 'The reason I'm upset about this is because I'm better than that. I'm going to get back on my workout routine tomorrow.' "

the coffee. You already know the dangers of too much caffeine. But bagging the most important meal of the day "can leave you dragging, and you can't be efficient if you're dragging at home, at work, or anywhere else," says Dr. Pace. If you're in a hurry, bring along at least a cup of low-fat yogurt, a piece of fruit, or even a bagel topped with a piece of low-fat cheese.

Lighten up lunch. Like to eat out at lunch? You're probably wasting a lot of valuable time getting there and waiting for service, says Dr. Pace. Not only that, but large, fat-laden lunches are guaranteed to slow you down later in the day, she says. Stick with lighter fare like salads with reduced-fat dressing, and lean sandwiches made with muscle-building protein like turkey, tuna, or chicken, and mustard and low-fat mayo.

Delay dinner. If you'd like to add another productive hour to your afternoon (for a workout, perhaps?) consider delaying dinner until 7:00 P.M., says Dr. Pace. This meal normally slows you down, "both in the time that you eat it and the effect it has on your mind and body," Dr. Pace says.

If you don't think you can make it that long without food, nosh on some manly snacks like popcorn, pretzels, or cereal.

Wake up. If you're getting more than seven hours of sleep each night, some experts suggest that you may be snoozing too much, says Dr. Pace. Here's the best way to gradually change that habit. Start waking up 15 minutes earlier every two weeks until you've reached your limit. And don't try going to bed later—that will only turn you into a sleepyhead, she says. And of course, early-morning hours are a prime time to hit the gym or the road for a run.

Get quality shut-eye. Caffeine, alcohol, and over-the-counter medications are notorious for preventing quality sleep, says Dr. Pace. Caffeine can disrupt sleep for up to five hours after you've had a slug; alcohol

Office Max

It seems that no matter what you do, you always get stuck at the office later than you'd like. And more often than not, it winds up eating into *your* time, including your exercise time. What you need is some practical advice on how to get out of the office at least an hour sooner. Meet Jeffrey J. Mayer, author of *If You Haven't Got the Time to Do It Right, When Will You Find the Time to Do It Over?* and *Time Management for Dummies*.

"My whole theme is this: Let's convert wasted time into time you can use more productively—like a workout," Mayer says. Here are some of Mayer's best tips to help you get it done and get to the gym.

Make appointments with yourself. "This is the number one time-saving tip. Appointments with yourself are nonnegotiable. If you have work to do and the boss assigned you a project, and it's going to take two hours, schedule it on your calendar as a nonnegotiable, noncancelable meeting that can't be interrupted for anything. And then get it done," says Mayer. You should plan workout sessions in the same way and keep them, he says.

Clear the clutter. Let's start by making one thing perfectly clear: your desk. Those huge stacks of so-called important papers? Lose 'em. Now. When you're done, Mayer says, "your desk should look like the flight deck of

dramatically reduces the amount of time that you spend in your natural deep-sleep cycle, she says. It's the same for many over-the-counter medications. And when you're groggy the next day, it's hard to function efficiently—which can translate into late-night work sessions and skipped workouts.

Cash in automatically. It feels nice to visit the pay window every Friday and collect your green, but it means driving to the bank,

an aircraft carrier. Most people leave stuff out on their desk as reminders of things to do, thinking that if they see it, they'll remember to do it. But it doesn't work. The stuff gets lost or buried and is forgotten, and it remains forgotten until someone wants it from you."

File those piles. All those papers go into just one of two places: file folders that are then placed in drawers, or the circular file. And remember: If you're going to win the battle against clutter, this is no time to get sentimental.

"Realistically, 60 percent of the stuff on your desk can go," says Mayer. "And about 80 percent of what's already in your file drawer can be tossed. If you do it right, you're left with only a handful of things that are really important."

Make a master list. In place of all those piles—and even the ever-popular notes stuck all over your office— place a large, clean sheet of lined paper on your newly immaculate desk and list all the things that you need to do, one item per line.

"The idea is that instead of leaving things out on the desktop as a reminder of things to do, why not put things on a list and get rid of the piles?" says Mayer. If you're a computer user, there are programs that work just as well, says Mayer. Cross off each item on the master list with a big line when it's completed.

more time to spend in the gym. If, that is, you can afford the membership after paying your bills.

Do two things at once. Okay, it's Saturday morning and you're dying to work out, but you have to take your kid to soccer practice—and the gym is on the other side of town. Why not root for your budding Pelé for a half-hour and then run, walk, or jog around the athletic field for a half-hour? Or suppose you need to go to the dry cleaner. Is there anything you need from the bank or store on the way as well? It may seem obvious, but stacking errands can shave minutes—even hours—off your schedule. Keep a to-do list on your fridge so that you can remember what needs to be done next.

Have some reading handy. Since surveys show that the average executive spends 15 minutes a day on hold, it pays to have some reading handy. May we suggest a certain magazine or workout/time-management book that can help you plan a more efficient workout strategy?

Dial on the wild side. Abandon your telephone technophobia. If we can learn how to use speed dial, you can, too. Because instructions differ from phone to phone, we can't detail them here. But just think how much time you'll save if you don't have to look up certain numbers, misdial, or have to redial.

Plug in. Are you still the only person on your block without a cordless phone, call waiting, a fax or answering machine, or a personal computer? Join the twentieth century—while there's still time—and buy or lease them. Some may argue that these devices actually steal time by keeping you constantly linked to work. But how many times have you been forced to drive to a print shop to send a fax when you could have been mountain biking or taking a dip?

filling out a deposit slip, and getting stuck in line behind some clown juggling 10 transactions. If your company has direct deposit, sign up and let them handle it for you. And while you're at it, you might want to take advantage of paying your bills automatically. Just about everyone from mortgage companies to the folks at your friendly, neighborhood public utility offers this service for free. Why? It won't take you as long to pay bills, and that means that you'll have

Keys to Motivation

Practical Tips to Stay Focused

Zig Ziglar, motivational speaker and author extraordinaire, lacking in motivation? When it comes to exercise, sometimes, truthfully, the answer is yes.

"On those days—which come often—that is where the word *discipline* enters the picture," Ziglar says. "I have already made a decision. This is what I'm going to do. And then on those days when you are kind of dragging, you do not make a new decision, because it will be an emotional decision when you are at a low ebb. Stick with the original decision, and take the first few minutes of exercise out of sheer willpower and commitment. And the rest of the exercise will just take care of itself—once you get those endorphins and dopamine and epinephrine hopping in your system."

Take It from the Pros

In addition to Ziglar, we spoke to personal trainers at some of the finest fitness facilities in the country and asked them to share some of their secrets for getting or staying motivated about exercise. Here's what they said.

Get real. Hands down, setting realistic goals was most commonly cited as the number one motivator. "Rather than pledging to work out two hours a day for the rest of your life, shoot for two or three one-hour training sessions a week at the beginning," says Courtney Barroll, a certified personal trainer and medical exercise specialist at Equinox Fitness Club in New York City. "The people

who go super gung ho in the beginning are usually the fastest to burn out. But they're setting themselves up for that. I think extremism leads to burnout. Moderation is the key to long-term success."

Allow a day off. If you miss one or more workouts, you basically have two choices. You can give yourself a mental body slam, draining any remaining motivation you may have. Or you can recognize that it takes weeks to lose your progress and that as soon as you get back in the gym, you'll be back on track. Guess which is better?

"For some reason missing a day or two has such strong ramifications psychologically that people almost feel like, 'I'm a loser. This isn't worth it,' " Barroll says. "But it's easy to get back on track. Take one day at a time. Missing a day or two is healthy. The body needs to recover. Don't look at it as a setback."

See the muscle. Some bodybuilders expose their weakest body part in the gym, hoping that seeing it—and any ribbing they get (example: Are those your calves, or are you walking on stilts?)—will motivate them to train harder. That can be counterproductive. It makes much more sense to wear clothes that reveal some of your progress. That will serve as a visible reminder that your hard work is paying off.

"I definitely think that it's a motivator to see those muscles emerging when you're working out," Barroll says.

Quit the comparisons. "This isn't a contest. Instead of comparing yourself to a great body across the gym, channel that energy into your own workout," says Barroll.

Do what you like. Has someone talked you into a super intense running program that's more likely to make you vomit than achieve a new personal best? Skip it—and stick with what you like, says Barroll. "If I put clients on machines that they aren't happy with or give them exercises that they don't like, they're going to be uncomfortable, and that's a de-motivator. If you hate the treadmill and love the bicycle, do the bike. And don't let anyone tell you otherwise. The object is to get people to like exercise, not dread it."

Play your song. When it looked like Rocky was going to get pounded by that huge Russian guy, did he surrender? Heck, no! He trained like a maniac to the orchestral strains of his very own theme song. Now there might be a few guys out there who never get tired of training, but the rest of us aren't too proud to admit the sad truth: Sometimes working out is downright boring.

On those days, it pays to let your favorite music motivate you. All you need are six or seven great songs to get you through the most painful 20-minute cardiovascular routine, says Marc Goodman, a fitness instructor and personal trainer at Crunch, a gym in New York City. What to choose? Your favorites, of course. And make sure that they're upbeat. Ours? *The Rocky Story*—a compact disc that contains hits from the movies. "Eye of the Tiger," baby.

Pick a partner. Like the Good Book says, "As iron sharpens iron, so one man sharpens another." Nothing motivates us more than a training partner focused on results. For best results—if your ego can handle it—try to find one who's stronger and more knowledge-able than you, suggests Steven Wheelock, fitness co-director of Canyon Ranch Lifestyle Resort in Lenox, Massachusetts. "Keeping up will be a challenge, but you'll definitely learn and grow," he says.

Picture success. Visualization—forming mental images of yourself doing some-thing successfully—has been proven effective by research. In one such study, basketball players were divided into two groups: those who weren't to practice at all and those who were instructed to visualize the ball swishing through the net over and over. When both groups returned to the court, the guys who saw their success sank significantly more baskets than the others. (Obviously, former NBA great Wilt Chamberlain had his mind on other things besides sinking free throws.)

"And, although it's a great motivator, this doesn't just apply to sports. You can use it in a tough business situation, challenging relation-ship issues—whenever you need results," says Rebecca Gorrell, a certified exercise leader and wellness education director at Canyon Ranch Fitness Resort in Tucson, Arizona.

Just make sure that the image you're choosing is realistic for your potential. "You want to try to improve on your genetic framework, not someone else's," says Barroll.

Pick the right place. Unless you're in-dependently wealthy, laying out the cash to join a gym will, theoretically, motivate you to show up. But you may find more excuses not to go if you've chosen a place to exercise that you don't really like. Prefer sweat, blood, and lots of grunting? Obviously, an aerobics studio isn't for you. Like to jog on the beach? Then why are you running around the track? says Barroll.

Tailor your workouts. Remember when you used to fill out your letterman jacket in all the right places? Striving to repeat that pleasant past can help motivate you to keep ex-ercising. Or promise to buy yourself a new Ar-mani suit when the shoulders and chest on this one get too small. "You might think that this just works for women, but I have male clients who talk about this, too," says Goodman.

Mix it up. Performing the same exercise routines month after month can make you feel like you're an automaton in a weight-lifting fac-tory. Instead, try to incorporate new exercises, machines, and equipment into every workout, says Wheelock.

"I think that this is one of the best ways to keep yourself motivated. And there are a mil-lion things that you can do. We have one class here where we put out 15 different weight sta-tions and have the guests train for a minute on the treadmill," he says. "Then we blow a whistle and they go to a weight station and do that for 45 seconds. They go back and forth be-tween the treadmill and the weights for all 15 different stations. It only takes 30 minutes, but you're combining aerobic and strength training.

Best of all, it's something different."

Get bitten by the competition bug.
If you got your last taste of athletic competition on a high school or college field—and have been sitting on the sidelines ever since— planning to enter a race or sports contest could be your motivational ticket, Wheelock says.

"We don't want to tell people to go out and jump into a biathlon or triathlon, but a charity run, walk, or jog definitely gives you something to train for," says Wheelock. "You start thinking: 'I have a race in August, and I'm going to put some time into it to get ready.' "

Not only that, but many events are held to raise money for charity. "It makes you feel good, and it's a good environment to be around," Wheelock says.

Turn up the intensity. We all know that the no-pain, no-gain philosophy to exercise can get us into trouble. But intense exercise does often lead to a kind of soreness that dedicated gym-goers crave. "It's like a Red Badge of Courage for your effort," Gorrell says. "You don't want to feel that way all the time. And for someone who is just starting out, it may actually be de-motivating. But for the rest of us, it's a feeling we look forward to that lets us know we're in the zone."

If you want to limit muscle soreness your first few times at the gym, stick with just one set of each exercise and use light weights for no more than 12 reps, Gorrell says.

Fight the feeling. Your training results are just a few weeks away, but you feel like your motivation is flagging. What to do? Educate yourself. Go to a bookstore and study fitness magazines or books, or talk to others in the gym who look like they know what they're doing. It may go against every Y chromosome that you have, but you'll probably learn something.

"I've found that people who are involved in fitness or have a passion for it are very willing to share info. Get into the more technical aspects of the training," says Gorrell. "Just don't let someone talk you into something crazy."

Chart your progress. A log that you bring and update while you exercise will help remind you where you've been—and where you're going. "Aside from the exercise and the numbers of sets and reps, you can write down how things felt, what was difficult, and what you need to do more of," Gorrell suggests.

Get a fix on your flab. Not the bookkeeping type? There's another way—if you don't mind letting a stranger pinch your soft spots. It's called a body composition analysis and just about any gym with a pair of skinfold calipers can do the trick. By measuring the skinfold thickness (the amount of fat right under your skin) at your shoulder blade, waist, back of your calf, biceps, triceps, or front of your thigh, you'll know your body's muscle-to-fat ratio. Before the session is over, schedule another pinch-a-thon six months later.

"You can imagine how motivating it would be to reduce your body fat and increase your muscle mass over time," Gorrell says.

Face the fear. If you'd like to train for a triathlon but swim like a stone, consider hitting the pool first. "Facing the fear is probably going to provide more juice than anything else," says Joe Ogilvie, a fitness leader at Chelsea Piers Sports and Entertainment Center in New York City. "Once you discover that you can do it, you'll be motivated to improve in other areas as well."

Take a class. If you've never explored the wide world of exercise, learning a little about a particular area can be a great motivator. Many gyms and fitness centers offer everything from karate and aeroboxing to nature walks and triathlon training. "It's much easier to get excited about something when it's approachable and less imposing," Ogilvie says.

Celebrate small victories. Just stepping foot on the jogging track may be a major accomplishment for some; others may have worked for what seemed like months to trim just a few seconds off their best 10-K time. Either way, give yourself credit for these accomplishments—they're the stepping-stones to future success, says Ogilvie.

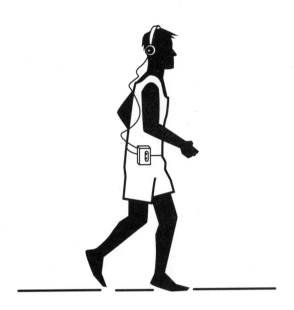

Part Two

Doing It Right

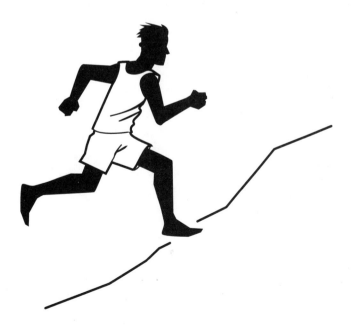

The Core Weight Workout

Like John Wayne said, a man's gotta do what a man's gotta do. And when it comes to resistance training, there are just some exercises that you can't afford to leave out of your workout program—even if you are in a hurry.

To find out which exercises belong on the can't-miss list, we turned to John Abdo, certified strength and conditioning specialist and host of the syndicated fitness television show *Training and Nutrition 2000,* and Bob Lefavi, Ph.D., a sports nutrition and strength-training specialist at Armstrong Atlantic State University in Savannah, Georgia, and the 1990 International Federation of Bodybuilding North American bantamweight bodybuilding champion.

What follows are their recommendations for the best weight-training exercises for

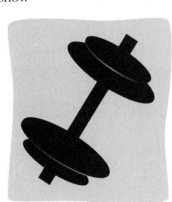

strengthening and building muscle in the shortest amount of time. Most of these exercises allow you to work several muscle groups at once, providing more muscular bang for your workout buck.

Of course, you'll get the best muscle-building gains if you can perform three sets for 8 to 12 repetitions. But if you're pinched for time, performing one set with a moderately heavy weight for 12 to 20 reps is a solid alternative. Under this one-set scenario, if it takes you about a minute to perform each exercise and you rest and shoot the breeze for a minute between sets, you'll be hitting the showers just 20 minutes from now, muscles pumped.

Prefer to do three sets? You'll need an hour to get it all done. Later in this section, you'll find complete workouts for whatever time you can spare— from 10 minutes to 90 minutes. The workouts will be drawn from the following exercises, along with those in the following two illustrated chapters: The Core Weightless Workout and The Ultimate 10-Minute Ab Workout.

Chest, Shoulders, Triceps, Biceps
Bench Press

Lie on your back on a bench with the barbell above your chest with a wider-than-shoulder-width grip. Keep your feet flat on the floor.

Slowly lower the barbell to your nipple line. Without bouncing the weight off your chest or lifting your butt off the bench, push the barbell back to arms' length.

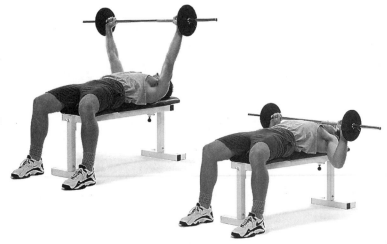

Upper Chest, Shoulders, Triceps
Inclined Bench Press

Lie on your back on an inclined bench-press apparatus set at an angle of 15 to 35 degrees. Grasp the bar with your palms up and your hands slightly wider than shoulder-width apart. Take the weight off the rack so that your arms are perpendicular to the floor.

Lower the bar to a point on your chest two inches below the clavicle area—commonly referred to as the collarbone—of your upper chest. Try to keep your elbows away from your torso. Raise the bar to the starting point, hold briefly, and repeat.

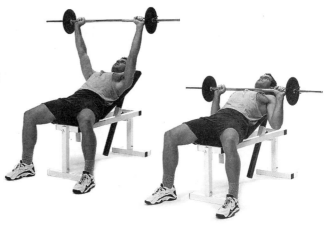

Upper Back (Lats and Traps), Rear Shoulders, Biceps
Barbell Bent-Over Rows

With a bar on the floor in front of you and your feet roughly shoulder-width apart, grasp the bar palms down so that your hands are about 24 to 26 inches from each other. Keep a slight bend in your knees, and maintain a natural curve in your lower back. Raise your torso so that your upper body is parallel to the floor, and keep your arms straight. The weight should come off the floor and not touch the floor again until the set is over.

Pull the bar upward so that it touches your chest at the bottom of your pectoral muscles (the very top of your abdomen). Hold momentarily, lower the bar to the starting position, and repeat.

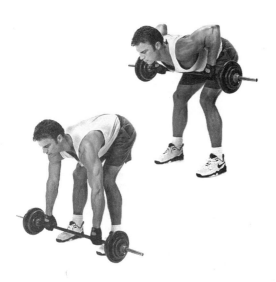

Back, Shoulders, Arms
Front Lat Pull-Downs

Sit at a lat pull-down machine and reach up, using a moderately wide grip to grab the bar. Look up slightly to tilt your head back.

Pull the bar down to your collarbone. Resist the weight as it goes back up. For the best gains, concentrate on squeezing your shoulder blades together as you perform the movement.

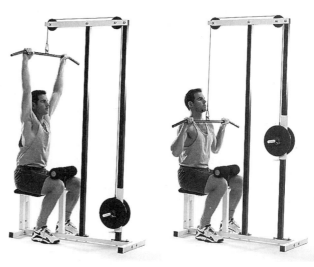

Triceps
Seated Overhead Triceps Extensions

Sit on a bench with your feet firmly on the ground and a dumbbell held overhead, palms facing up. Your upper torso should be erect and facing forward, with a slight natural forward lean in your lower back.

Keeping your upper body in place, lower the dumbbell behind your head. Keep your upper arms close to your head, and lower the dumbbell in a semicircular motion until your forearms are as close to your biceps as possible. You might lean slightly forward to help offset the weight, but don't sway or arch your back. Your elbows should be facing forward. Raise to the starting position.

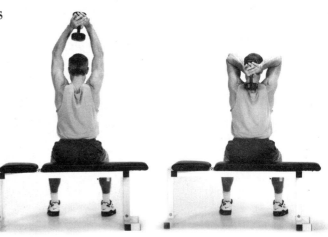

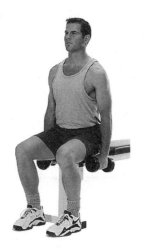
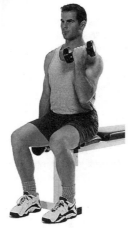

Biceps, Forearms
Seated Dumbbell Curls

Sit on a bench holding a dumbbell in each hand. Your back should be upright, and your palms facing in.

Slowly curl the weight in your left hand. As the dumbbell passes your thigh, twist your hand and wrist, rotating your thumb outward. For added benefit, flex your bicep at the top. Lower the weight slowly, reversing the rotation on the way down, and repeat with the other arm.

Shoulders, Triceps
Seated Military Press

Sit on the end of a bench, with your feet firmly planted on the floor. Hold a barbell across the front of your shoulders with your palms facing out, hands slightly wider than shoulder-width apart. Sit up straight, with your shoulders, back, and chest slightly out.

Without rocking or swaying to gain momentum, push the barbell above your head until your arms are fully extended. Lower the weight.

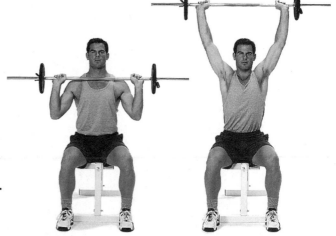

Shoulders, Upper Back, Biceps, Forearms
Upright Rows

Stand upright holding a barbell in both hands, your palms down in a narrow grip. Your arms should be fully extended in front of you, the barbell at your upper thighs. Allow your shoulders to relax slightly, but keep your back straight.

Pull the barbell straight up, and tuck it under your chin. Your elbows should be pointing up and out. Hold briefly and lower the weight.

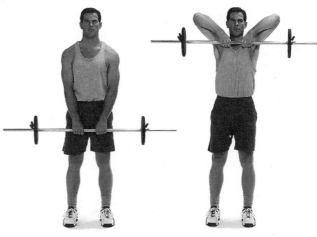

Quadriceps, Hips, Buttocks, Back, Calves
Back Squats

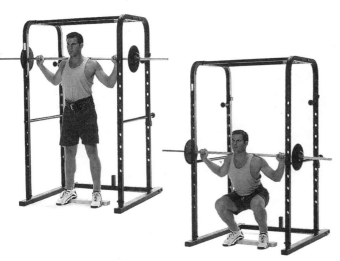

Lay a two-by-four two steps in front of a squat rack. Stand before the squat rack, grasping the bar palms down. Dip your head and step under the bar until it rests just below your neck and across your upper back. Lift the bar with your legs and carefully step backward until your heels rest shoulder-width apart on the two-by-four.

With your head up, back straight, feet shoulder-width apart, and toes facing slightly outward, squat until your thighs are parallel to the floor. Exhale as you press your body up. Do not lean forward. Use a belt to support the lower back.

Lower Back, Hamstrings, Buttocks
Stiff-Legged Dead Lifts

Stand with your feet shoulder-width apart, with a barbell on the floor in front of you (the bar should be over your feet and close to your shins). Keeping your back straight, your head up, and your shoulders directly over or a little ahead of the bar, squat down and grasp the bar with your arms extended and positioned just outside your knees. One palm should face out, the other palm in.

Stand up holding the bar, raising it straight up off the floor, using your thighs and back, keeping your arms extended and back straight. Once upright, lower the weight back to the floor again.

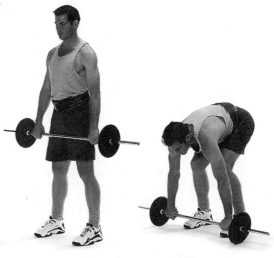

The Core Weightless Workout

You don't have to invest in a gym membership or an Olympic weight set to build muscle. All you need is some rubber exercise tubing, common office furniture, and determination.

"For guys out there who are thinking, 'There's no rubber band out there that can challenge me!' I can tell you that we've done studies that show that these work for even the strongest of men," says Alan Mikesky, Ph.D., an exercise physiologist and director of the Human Performance and Biochemistry Laboratory at Indiana University-Purdue University in Indianapolis. "And the great part is that they weigh next to nothing and take virtually no space. You can throw them in your suitcase and take them on the road."

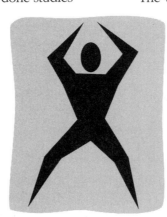

The weightless exercises that follow are recommended by certified strength and conditioning specialist John Abdo and Armstrong Atlantic State University's Dr. Bob Lefavi.

"This goes against the traditional thinking, which says that you have to go into a gym and lift a heavy weight for eight reps to gain muscle," Abdo says. "But if you look at skaters or swimmers or rowers or boxers who do hundreds of sports-specific movements, most people would agree they have well-built physiques. Whatever exercise you are doing, if you take that muscle past its normal rep range and push beyond that—even without weights—you are going to see increases in muscular development."

The weightless exercises that follow should be performed as many times as possible until you experience muscular fatigue, Abdo says.

"You push until you can't do any more. Then you stop," he says. "You don't sit there for three seconds and then try to squeeze out more repetitions. If you have to pause three or more seconds, the set is over with. The muscle has failed at that point, and that was the objective—to bring the muscle to failure."

Chest, Shoulders, Triceps
Push-Ups between Chairs

Position two sturdy chairs far enough from a bed or bench so that you can place your feet onto the bed and each hand shoulder-width apart on each of the two chairs. The chairs must be spread apart enough for your chest to fit between them. Get into the starting position with your legs and back rigid and your arms vertical to the floor.

Slowly bend your elbows, lowering your chest until it descends below the level of your hands on the two chairs. Pause, then press back to the starting position. Repeat.

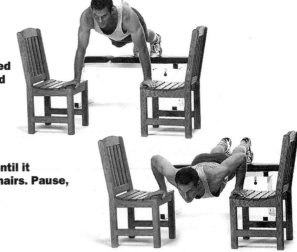

Chest, Shoulders, Triceps
Decline Push-Ups

Kneel on the floor in front of a flat bench or table with your hands shoulder-width apart and under your chest. Place your feet on the bench or table behind you.

With your back straight and head up, lower yourself until your chest slightly touches the floor. Pause at the bottom, then press back to the starting position. Repeat.

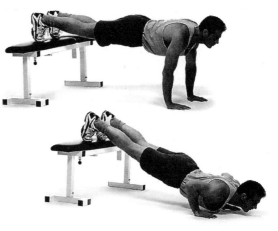

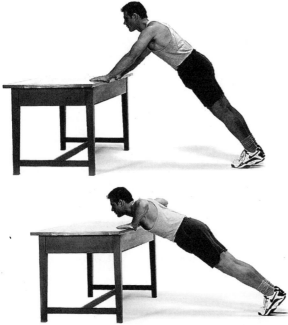

Chest, Shoulders, Triceps
Desk Push-Ups

Place your hands slightly wider than shoulder-width apart on the front edge of a sturdy desk. Straighten your arms and step back until your body forms a 45-degree angle with the floor. Your weight is resting on your hands and the balls of your feet.

Keeping your legs and back rigid, slowly bend your elbows until your chest slightly touches the desk. Push back to the starting position. Repeat.

Upper Back, Rear Shoulders, Biceps, Lower Back
Seated Two-Arm Rows

Sit on the floor with your legs straight in front of you, feet pointing up. Place the rubber exercise tubing around your feet and grasp it by the handles. Your arms should be extended straight in front of you, and your back should be upright.

Pull the tubing toward your chest, squeezing your shoulder blades together as you move. Return the tubing to the starting position and repeat.

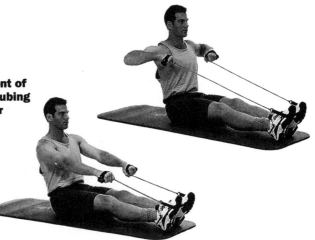

Triceps
Desk Dips

Stand with your back toward a sturdy desk, and your palms braced on the edge just outside the width of your buttocks. Move your feet forward until your buttocks just clear the edge of the desk. Support your weight on your heels.

Slowly bend your elbows, lowering your buttocks toward the floor until your elbows are bent at 90 degrees. Push yourself back up to the starting position. Repeat.

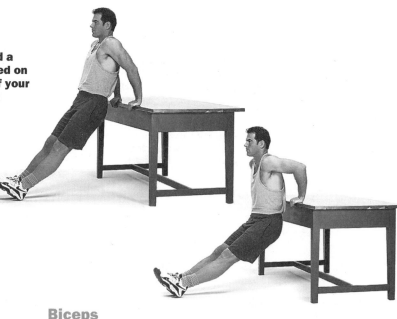

Biceps
Biceps Curls

With your feet spread shoulder-width apart, hook some exercise tubing under each foot and grasp the handles.

With your arms at your sides and palms facing in, slowly curl your right arm up, keeping your right elbow against your side. As your right hand passes your thigh, twist your wrist so your palm faces up. Continue curling until your hand reaches shoulder height. Slowly lower and repeat with your left hand.

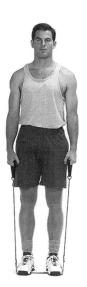
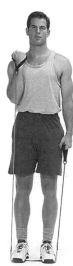

Shoulders, Triceps, Biceps, Forearms
Upright Rows

While standing upright with the rubber exercise tubing under your feet, grasp the handles with your palms facing toward your body. Pull the tubing up, leading with your elbows.

Bring the tubing up until your hands are tucked under your chin. (Keep your elbows out as you perform the movement.) Slowly lower the tubing and repeat.

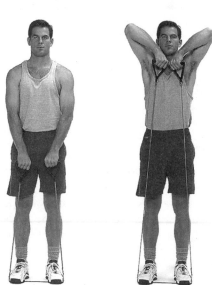

Quadriceps, Hamstrings, Buttocks, Hips, Back
Squats

Stand upright with your feet shoulder-width apart and your toes pointed slightly outward. Your arms should be straight out in front of you for balance, with palms facing down. Keep your back straight.

Squat down until your thighs are parallel with the floor. Keep your back straight through the motion, using your arms for balance. Press yourself back to the standing upright position. Rather than hesitating between reps, you should look like a piston pumping up and down. Feel free to shift your feet wider or narrower to isolate different portions of your leg muscles and re-duce fatigue on others.

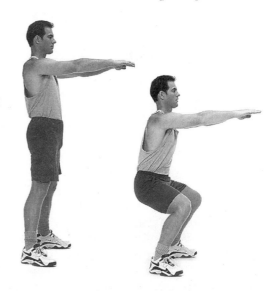

Quadriceps, Hips, Hamstrings, Inner Thighs, Buttocks, Calves
Front Lunges

Stand upright, with your hands on your hips or clasped behind your head.

Keeping your back straight, step forward with your right foot until your right thigh is parallel with the floor. Push back to the starting position, then repeat with your left leg. Repeat.

Calves, Achilles Tendons
Heel-Ups

Stand upright with the pads of your left foot on the edge of a step or raised object a few inches off the ground. Wrap your right foot around and behind your left ankle.

With your back straight, raise your left heel as high as possible, pushing down with your toes. Hold that position for two seconds, then lower your heel slowly. Repeat with the opposite leg.

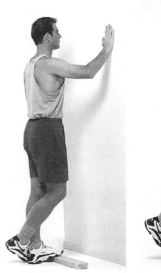
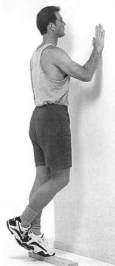

The Ultimate 10-Minute Ab Workout

They're the Holy Grail of fitness: washboard abs. But with your schedule, you're lucky to find time to get your wash done, let alone trying to deflate a bulging belly.

We sympathize with your dilemma, friend. That's why, with the help of certified strength and conditioning specialist John Abdo, we've created this 10-minute, foolproof, gut-busting plan—an exercise routine that, performed daily, will not only strengthen your waist but also carve in those cuts.

"I take an athletic approach to abdominal training," Abdo says. "So many athletes need to bend, twist, pivot, and rotate their torsos during their sports. These exercises and those that I've developed for my exercise video *Waste to Waist* were initially designed to improve the functionality of your torso, which includes your abdominals, obliques, and lower back. But these sports-training principles

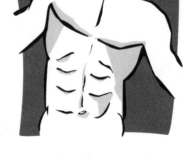

also manifest themselves as cosmetic benefits. That means that not only can you perform or function better but also your entire midsection starts looking terrific."

Before you begin, however, keep a couple of things in mind. You'll get the best burn if you do these exercises in sequence. And forget counting reps. Simply perform each for 30 seconds and, after a brief rest, move to the next. (All but the side oblique crunch and the arm and leg reach; these should be performed for 30 seconds each side.) After working through all the exercises, go back and select four favorites that train your upper abs, lower abs, obliques, and lower back.

Unless you're in great shape, chances are good that you'll have trouble performing these exercises for 10 minutes. But stay with it—that's the goal. If you don't have that much time to train your waist, just make sure that you select exercises that train all four areas. To freshen your routine after you're stronger, try performing the exercises in different order.

Go slow if you've never exercised before or have had lower-back or other health problems. And no matter how much you exercise, don't expect to sport a "six-pack" if you're drinking too many six-packs or eating a high-fat diet.

Okay, it's crunch time.

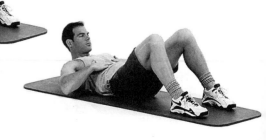

Upper Abdominals
Crunches

Lie on your back with your knees bent, feet flat on the floor, and hands touching your upper abs.

Using only your upper-abdominal muscles, curl your chest up a few inches until your shoulder blades are slightly off the floor. Hold briefly, lower, and repeat.

Lower Abdominals, Hips
V-Sits

Sit on the edge of a flat bench with your knees bent, and hold on to the sides.

Slowly pull your knees up toward your chest, contracting your lower abdominals. Hold briefly, then lower your legs and repeat.

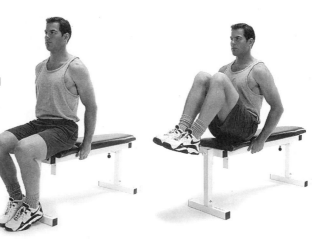

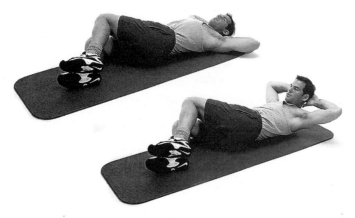

Obliques, Upper Abs
Side Oblique Crunches

Lie on your back with your hands behind your head and your legs bent to your right side, keeping your upper body flat on the floor.

Lift your shoulders and chest only a few inches off the ground, squeezing your left oblique muscles as you move. Lower and repeat. Switch sides and repeat.

Lower Abdominals, Hips
Reverse Crunches

Lie on the floor with your hands palms down under your lower back for support, knees bent, and feet flat on the floor.

Slowly pull your knees toward your chest and shoulders, curling your midsection and lifting your pelvis and buttocks off the floor, keeping your mid-to-upper back pressed against the floor. Slowly return to the starting position and repeat.

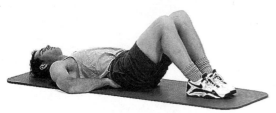

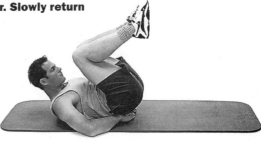

Obliques, Lower Back, Upper Abs
Seated Side Bends

While sitting upright on the floor, spread your legs as far apart as possible. Lift your chest up so that your back is straight, and lock your arms behind your head.

Lean a few inches to your right side, then swing over to the left. Continue pivoting like a pendulum, while trying to tense your stomach muscles.

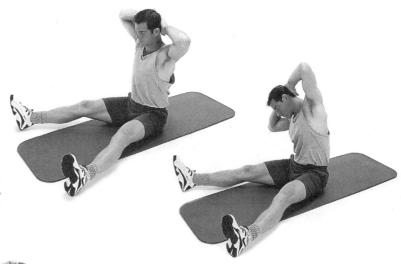

Upper and Lower Abdominals
Jackknife Sit-Ups

Lie on your back, placing your arms on the floor straight over your head.

Bending at the waist and balancing on your buttocks, simultaneously raise your arms and legs until your hands and feet meet like a jackknife. Lower your arms and legs.

Caution: **Do not attempt this exercise if you have back problems.**

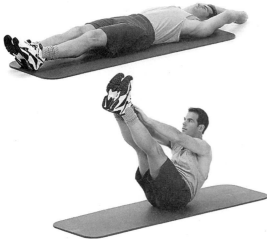

Obliques, Lower Back, Upper Abs, Lower Abs
Oblique Twists

Sit upright on the floor with your knees bent. Chin and chest should both be up.

Lean slightly rearward, then start twisting your torso from right to left with short pivots like you are performing a slow jog with your upper body. Use your arms to set a good tempo. Keep performing these twists until the set expires.

Caution: **Do not attempt this exercise if you have back problems.**

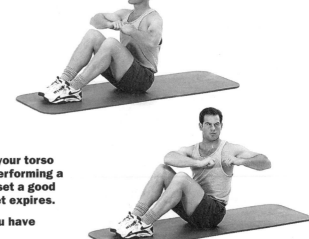

Lower to Middle Abdominals, Hips
Vertical Leg Lifts

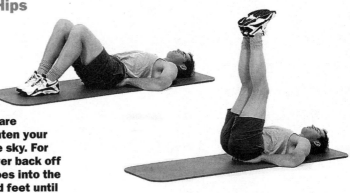

Lie on your back with your knees bent, feet flat on the ground, and your hands palms down under the small of your back.

Pull your knees in the direction of your chest until your thighs are perpendicular with the floor, then straighten your lower legs by lifting your feet toward the sky. For added benefit, lift your buttocks and lower back off the ground as if you are pressing your toes into the air. Slowly lower your buttocks, legs, and feet until you make contact with the floor, then repeat.

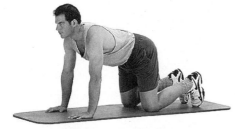

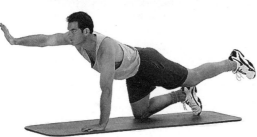

Lower Back, Mid-to-Upper Back, Buttocks
Arm and Leg Reaches

This exercise is necessary to isolate the rear portion of your lower back, a significant and often overlooked part of your midsection. Place hands and knees on the floor.

Reach with your right arm while simultaneously pushing your left leg back. Hold your arm and leg momentarily in their upright position, tensing all of your back and buttocks muscles, focusing mostly on your lower back, spinal muscles, and rear portion of your midsection. Perform this action without touching your right hand or left knee to the floor until you have completed all the reps for that side. Rest only a few seconds, then repeat with the left arm and right leg.

Obliques, Lower Back
Twisting Reaches

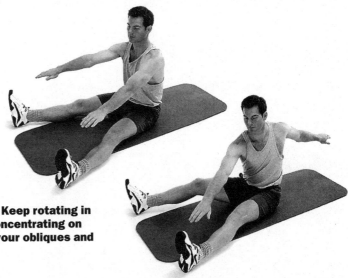

Sit upright and spread your legs as far apart as comfortable.

Straighten your back by lifting your chest, then rotate your torso to the left so your right hand reaches for your left foot. Rotate to the opposite side reaching now with your left hand for your right foot. Keep rotating in this pivot fashion until your set expires, concentrating on using all of your midsection—particularly your obliques and lower back—to drive your movement.

The Ultimate Fat-Burning Workout

Like Tim Allen's character on *Home Improvement*, constantly looking to turbocharge the vacuum, lawn mower, and toaster oven, guys naturally believe that more power is always better. Well, that's not always so, especially when it comes to fitness. Sometimes making like an iron man isn't the best course of action—especially if your goal is to burn fat.

That's because research indicates that working harder might actually leave you fatter. "One study found that walking at about 3.8 miles per hour (mph) for half an hour burned 240 calories, 40 percent of which was fat," says Wayne Westcott, Ph.D., of Quincy, Massachusetts, a strength-training consultant to the YMCA. "Running at 6.5 mph for that same half-hour burned 450 calories . . . however, only 25 percent of them were from fat." Slow, easy, relaxed—effective.

The reason is that the harder you exercise, the faster you need energy. And the high-carbohydrate snack you ate before exercising is far more easily metabolized than the layers of "greaseburgers" and lager you've been carrying around for years. To burn that off, you have to retrofit your fat incinerator.

Increase Intensity

The key to burning fat is interval training. Consider a study conducted at Laval University in Sainte Foy, Quebec, where researchers measured differences in fat loss between two groups of exercisers following two different workout programs. The first group pedaled stationary bikes four or five times a week for a moderate burn of 300 to 400 calories per 30- to 45-minute session.

The second group did the same, but only one or two times a week, and they filled in the rest of their sessions with short intervals of high-intensity cycling: They hopped on their stationary bikes and pedaled as quickly as they could for 30 to 90 seconds, rested, and then repeated the process several times per exercise session.

As a result, these slackers burned only about 225 to 250 calories while cycling. But they also burned more fat by the end of the study than the hard workers in group one. In fact, their fat loss was *nine times greater.*

Researchers offer a theory about what happened to the second group. "It's true that during the actual workout, the harder you exercise, the more likely it is that your body will preferentially burn carbohydrates over fat," says study leader Angelo Tremblay, Ph.D., professor of physiology and nutrition at Laval University. "But eventually, after the workout is over, your body has to replace the calories that it used. We think that the fat-reduction effect occurs after the exercise."

High-intensity interval training, anyone? While the jury is still out pending additional research, Dr. Tremblay suggests that short-term, high-intensity training may encourage the body to find lost calories by pillaging fat stores to a greater degree than it would after moderate exercise. And your body does it long after the last wind sprint is over.

"There are studies that show that the metabolism stays elevated for 15 hours after high-intensity strength training," says Dr. Westcott. So if you open your throttle for several 60- to 90-second intervals over the course of your workout, your fat burners may be turned up for nearly two-thirds of the day. And this is an exchange rate we can all live with.

But before we get started, we'll need to agree on a definition of *high-intensity*. Exercise is really intense if you're pedaling, running, or stair-climbing fast enough to make conversation difficult. To test yourself, try chanting the first three lines of your fave rock anthem at about the 60-second mark. If you can't make it to line two, you're in the target zone. If you can get through the first verse of "Layla" (acoustic version), you need to work harder. And you have to go hard for as long as you can, with 90 seconds as the goal. If you lower the intensity to last longer, your fat-burning inferno will die down to Zippo-lighter strength.

A Winning Combination

Okay, now we're going to up the ante. We want you to train using the interval method. And we want you to do it at the same time you're weight training.

There are two reasons. First, while the high-intensity interval trainers in the Laval University study did rest between their short bursts of activity, their heart rates never dropped below 120 beats per minute. Some light resistance training will make sure that yours doesn't either. Second, you'll add muscle, another fat burner.

"Muscle is more metabolically active than fat, so each pound of lean tissue you add means that you burn an extra 35 calories a day whether you are sitting, sleeping, or watching TV," says Dr. Westcott. Add three pounds of muscle to your frame and you can figure in about an extra pound of fat burned each month, without even trying.

Get with the Program

To make the principle of interval training work for you, take whatever kind of aerobic-exercise machine you have—a treadmill, stair-climber, stationary bike—and stick it in one room. Now pick up your resistance-training equipment—whether it's dumbbells, barbells, a machine, or just exercise tubing—and put them in an adjoining room. Of course, if you work out at a gym, they've already got things set up for you. The idea here is to move back and forth between the two forms of exercise so that you get a brief—maybe 10-second—cooling-off period between each activity.

Here's the program recommended by Armstrong Atlantic State University's Dr. Bob Lefavi.

Warm up. This is a strenuous workout, and the worst way to go about it is to explode from the starting block at top speed. Spend three to five minutes on a treadmill, bike, or steps moving at a slow to moderate pace. And the same advice applies when you're cooling down at the end of your workout.

Run like hell. After you've warmed up, continue treading, pedaling, or stepping; but pick up the pace to heart-pounding levels. You've just started the workout proper. Do this for either 30, 60, or 90 seconds (whatever you can manage initially).

Walk this way. Now stop, walk down the hall (permission to pant granted), and pick up the dumbbells for a round of resistance exercise.

Lift. Do one set of one resistance exercise. (For a suggested weight-training routine, see The Ultimate 30-Minute Workout, weight version, on page 52.) Now drop the weights, head back up the hall, and do the aerobics for another 90 seconds. Then back down the hall. Get the picture?

The suggested circuit includes seven resistance moves and eight aerobic bouts, which will take you about 20 minutes. Try to work up to twice around for a 40-minute workout. But be prudent. Do what you can.

If 20 minutes seems to be your limit, use the remaining 20 for moderate aerobic activity—light walking or comfortable stationary biking. Eventually, you'll find yourself extending the heavy-duty workout and cutting back on the light to moderate. And as you do, watch the fat fly . . . fly away, that is.

The Ultimate 10-Minute Workout

There will be days when you think that you simply don't have time to exercise. But that's rarely true. It's just that you don't have as much time as you'd like to exercise. Or you don't have enough time to do your full normal routine, whether it's walking, jogging, bicycling, lifting weights, or playing basketball. That's an important distinction to understand.

The question you should ask yourself on days like these is, Can you spare 10 minutes? If you can, you have time to work out. Efficiency is the byword in business today. How else to boost productivity with fewer people and shrinking resources? Your workout need not be any different.

When time and equipment are at a premium, you have to make do with what you have. The trick here is targeting your largest muscles for training—quadriceps, pectorals, latissimus dorsi—and allowing your smaller muscles to also benefit from indirect stimulation, says Armstrong Atlantic State University's Dr. Bob Lefavi. And with just 10 minutes for

training, there's no room for indecision.

"You're going to want to plan this out so that you have the equipment accessible and know exactly what you're going to do," Dr. Lefavi says.

The exercises that follow are recommended by Dr. Lefavi because they provide the most muscular bang for your workout buck. For example, Dr. Lefavi chose inclined bench presses over traditional flat bench presses for this routine. "You're able to train the more important clavicular fibers of the chest with the inclined bench press, but because you're at an angle, you're working the front deltoids and the triceps a little more," he says.

Skip the seated two-arm row if you don't have any exercise tubing, but if you want a full-body workout while you're on the road, it would be worth your while to pick some up, Dr. Lefavi says. (One tubing system, called the Lifeline Gym, weighs just two pounds and allows you to perform more than 25 different aerobic and toning exercises for your back, chest, arms, legs, and shoulders. Call 1-800-553-6633 for the location of the store nearest you that carries Lifeline or for more information.)

Because your warm-up time is limited here, perform all exercises carefully. And if you can, sneak in some postworkout stretching in the shower, as you get dressed, or when you're back in the office.

Weight ⚹ Workout

Warm-Up (1 minute)
Jumping jacks or jogging in place

Exercises (9 minutes)

Squats (two sets, 8 to 12 reps, 30 seconds between sets)

Inclined bench press (two sets, 8 to 12 reps, 15 to 20 seconds between sets)

Barbell rows (two sets, 8 to 12 reps, 15 to 20 seconds between sets)

Crunches (one set to failure)

Weightless ⚹ Workout

Warm-Up (1 minute)
Jumping jacks or jogging in place

Exercises (9 minutes)

Lunges (two sets, 10 to 15 reps, 30 seconds between sets)

Decline push-ups (two sets, 10 to 15 reps, 15 to 20 seconds between sets)

Seated two-arm rows with tubing (two sets, 8 to 12 reps, 15 to 20 seconds between sets)

Crunches (one set to failure)

The Ultimate 20-Minute Workout

Think of it. In less time than it takes one company to rush a pizza to your door, you can perform the following workout—a routine that will not only train nearly all of your major muscle groups but also increase your flexibility.

Better yet, skip the pizza and just do the workout. All you need is 20 minutes—time that even the busiest guy can usually find.

You'll notice that adding just 10 minutes to The Ultimate 10-Minute Workout gives you the opportunity to focus more direct effort on those all-important chest and shoulder muscles. In the weight workout, we've replaced the inclined bench press that provided all the chest and shoulder work in The Ultimate 10-Minute Workout with bench presses and seated military presses.

Having 20 minutes to train gives you yet another advantage: the opportunity to stretch. Not only does a warm-up followed by stretching help prepare your muscles for your workout, but those four minutes can also be used to focus and visualize the improvements in your body that you want to make, says Dr. Lefavi.

Weight ⚡ Workout

Warm-Up (2 minutes)
Walk on treadmill, ride a stationary bike, jump rope, or perform a similar activity for 2 minutes. (Remember that a true warm-up increases your body's core temperature 1°F, so try to break a light sweat during the warm-up.)

Stretch (2 minutes)
Stretch the muscles to be trained. (While stretching, mentally prepare for the workout, focus on how you will move from one exercise to the next, and so on.)

Exercises (14 minutes)

Bench press (one set, 8 to 12 reps)

Barbell rows (one set, 8 to 12 reps)

Seated military press (one set, 8 to 12 reps)

Barbell curls (one set, 10 to 15 reps)

Overhead triceps extensions (one set, 10 to 15 reps)

Squats (one set, 8 to 12 reps)

Crunches (one set to failure)

Cooldown (2 minutes)
Perform any activity that uses large, major muscle groups in a rhythmical, continuous fashion, such as bicycling.

Weightless ⚡ Workout

Warm-Up (2 minutes)
Walk on treadmill, ride a stationary bike, jump rope, or perform a similar activity for 2 minutes. (Remember that a true warm-up increases your body's core temperature 1°F, so try to break a light sweat during the warm-up.)

Stretch (2 minutes)
Stretch the muscles to be trained. (While stretching, mentally prepare for the workout, focus on how you will move from one exercise to the next, and so on.)

Exercises (14 minutes)

Push-ups between chairs (one set, 10 to 15 reps)

Seated two-arm rows with tubing (one set, 8 to 12 reps)

Desk dips (one set, 10 to 15 reps)

Biceps curls with tubing (one set, 8 to 12 reps)

Upright rows with tubing (one set, 8 to 12 reps)

Lunges (one set, 10 to 15 reps)

Crunches (one set to failure)

Cooldown (2 minutes)
Perform any activity that uses large, major muscle groups in a rhythmical, continuous fashion, such as bicycling.

The Ultimate 30-Minute Workout

If you hustled, you could probably use every piece of equipment in your gym in 30 minutes. But why add exercises when research shows that increasing sets boosts workout benefits—as well as saves time?

"There's ample evidence that two sets are about 50 percent better than one," says Armstrong Atlantic State University's Dr. Bob Lefavi. "The muscle fibers begin to get the deep stimulation that's needed for enhanced growth."

Not only that, but a 30-minute workout enjoys a sort of celebrity status in the world of exercise physiology. Research shows that that's the amount of continuous exercise needed to help reap health benefits such as lower blood pressure. Normally, those results don't apply to weight workouts—unless you pick up the pace and keep your heart rate in the 60 to 90 percent maximum range.

A typical circuit-training session features 12 exercises using weights that are 40 to 50 percent of your one-rep maximum. You perform each exercise for 30 seconds, rest for 30 seconds, and then exercise for another 30 seconds. The cycle is repeated three to five times. That's not exactly the way we've structured this program, but you can adapt it to suit your interests and needs, says Dr. Lefavi.

A brief cardiovascular cooldown like running, walking, or using a stair-climber helps aid recovery by promoting blood flow through the muscle and removing lactic acid. And that can help reduce delayed onset muscle soreness—a fancy name for the pain you may feel tomorrow, Dr. Lefavi says.

You may be wondering why Dr. Lefavi recommends squats as the only leg exercise in the weight workout, and lunges for the weightless workout. The reason is that lunges challenge the muscles of each leg individually.

Weight Workout

Warm-Up (3 minutes)

Walk on treadmill, ride a stationary bike, jump rope, or perform a similar activity for 3 minutes. (Remember that a true warm-up increases your body's core temperature 1°F, so try to break a light sweat during the warm-up.)

Stretch (2 minutes)

Stretch the muscles to be trained. (While stretching, mentally prepare for the workout, focus on how you will move from one exercise to the next, and so on.)

Exercises (22 minutes, with small amount of time allotted for weight adjustment)

Bench press (two sets, 8 to 12 reps, 1 minute between sets)

Barbell rows (two sets, 8 to 12 reps, 1 minute between sets)

Overhead triceps extensions (two sets, 10 to 15 reps, 45 seconds between sets)

Barbell curls (two sets, 10 to 15 reps, 45 seconds between sets)

Seated military press (two sets, 8 to 12 reps, 1 minute between sets)

Squats (two sets, 8 to 12 reps, 1 minute between sets)

Crunches (two sets, 15 to 30 reps, 1 minute between sets)

Cooldown (2 minutes)

Perform any activity that uses large, major muscle groups in a rhythmical, continuous fashion, such as bicycling.

Stretch (1 minute)

So if you don't have any weights handy, lunges isolate your glutes, hamstrings, quadriceps, and calves better than squats, Dr. Lefavi says. And that makes more effective use of your body weight for resistance. However, it's also tougher to keep your balance, and the movement requires more concentration to perform correctly.

Squats, on the other hand, can be done with heavier weights than lunges because the work is spread over both legs. That allows you to develop more explosive power, Dr. Lefavi says.

Note also that you're required to perform higher reps if you choose to do the weightless workout. "What you lack in intensity—weight—you need to make up in volume," Dr. Lefavi explains.

Building Aerobic Fitness

Three times a week, 52 weeks a year, you lift weights. But if you want to burn fat without tearing down your muscles while they're trying to repair, it's a good idea to work some aerobic activity into your weekly workouts, Dr. Lefavi says. True, you get a slight cardiovascular benefit from pumping iron. But once you manage to set aside 30 minutes a day for exercise, you have enough time to get the health benefits of moderate exercise recommended by that pesky Surgeon General. Plus, there's a good chance that aerobic exercise will help relieve any lingering muscle soreness from the squats and other exercises you did in yesterday's weight workout.

It's probably a good idea to limit your aerobic activity to two to three days that you aren't weight training, says Dr. Lefavi. Each of the following aerobic activities burns about 150 calories and shouldn't take more than 30 minutes to complete. Try:

- Bicycling five miles
- Running three miles
- Walking two miles

If you're concerned about possible injury from pounding the pavement while running, Dr. Lefavi recommends mixing up your aerobic activity. Try alternating between bicycling and running every couple of weeks.

Weightless 🏃 Workout

Warm-Up (3 minutes)

Walk, jump rope, or perform jumping jacks, squat thrusts, or similar activity for 3 minutes. (Remember that a true warm-up increases your body's core temperature 1°F, so try to break a light sweat during the warm-up.)

Stretch (2 minutes)

Stretch the muscles to be trained. (While stretching, mentally prepare for the workout, focus on how you will move from one exercise to the next, and so on.)

Exercises (22 minutes)

Push-ups between chairs (three sets, 10 to 15 reps, 45 seconds between sets)

Seated two-arm rows with tubing (three sets, 8 to 12 reps, 1 minute between sets)

Desk dips (two sets, 10 to 15 reps, 45 seconds between sets)

Biceps curls with tubing (two sets, 8 to 12 reps, 45 seconds between sets)

Upright rows with tubing (two sets, 8 to 12 reps, 1 minute between sets)

Lunges (three sets, 10 to 15 reps, 45 seconds between sets)

Crunches (two sets, 15 to 30 reps, 1 minute between sets)

Cooldown (2 minutes)

Perform any activity that uses large, major muscle groups in a rhythmical, continuous fashion, such as bicycling.

Stretch (1 minute)

The Ultimate 45-Minute Workout

Crank up the intensity. Not only does this training routine require three sets per exercise but we've also added a great new movement to your weight workout: the stiff-legged dead lift.

"The optimal volume—where you get the biggest bang for your exercise buck—is three sets," says Armstrong Atlantic State University's Dr. Bob Lefavi. "Plus, we're now hitting all the major muscle groups and have a few minutes more to hit them harder."

Don't get the wrong idea: One set works fine when you don't have the time. But three sets are tops for increasing strength and developing muscle.

In one study, researchers found that those volunteers who trained their legs for three sets over a 14-week period showed 15.5 percent strength gains, while those who did just one set per workout gained 14.5 percent. That doesn't seem like much of a difference—until you're under the weight and trying to drive it up.

Stiff-legged dead lifts will help develop your lower-back muscles, glutes, and hamstrings—areas that didn't get much attention in the shorter programs because of time constraints.

"You get lower-back activation in your squats. And you get some glute activation in your squats and lunges because of the hip extension, but you're not going to be able to work the hamstrings that well unless you do another exercise. But like a squat, the stiff-legged dead lift has the advantage of working several muscles simultaneously," he says. "It's a great exercise."

Until now we haven't said much about your ab work, but feel free to perform three different ab exercises—targeting different muscle groups—instead of simply doing three sets of

Weight Workout

Warm-Up (4 minutes)
Walk on a treadmill, ride a stationary bike, jump rope, or perform a similar activity for 4 minutes. (Remember that a true warm-up increases your body's core temperature 1°F, so try to break a light sweat during the warm-up.)

Stretch (3 minutes)
Stretch the muscles to be trained. (While stretching, mentally prepare for the workout, focus on how you will move from one exercise to the next, and so on.)

Exercises (33 minutes; with small amount of time allotted for weight adjustment)
Bench press (three sets, 8 to 12 reps, 1 minute between sets)

Barbell rows (three sets, 8 to 12 reps, 1 minute between sets)

Overhead triceps extensions (three sets, 10 to 15 reps, 45 seconds between sets)

Barbell curls (two sets, 10 to 15 reps, 45 seconds between sets)

Seated military press (three sets, 8 to 12 reps, 1 minute between sets)

Squats (three sets, 8 to 12 reps, 1 minute between sets)

Stiff-legged dead lifts (two sets, 10 to 15 reps, 1 minute between sets)

Crunches (three sets, 15 to 30 reps, 1 minute between sets)

Cooldown (3 minutes)
Perform any activity that uses large, major muscle groups in a rhythmical, continuous fashion, such as bicycling.

Stretch (2 minutes)

standard crunches. (You'll find 10 different ab exercises illustrated in The Ultimate 10-Minute Ab Workout on page 44.) In fact, since your body adapts quickly to muscular stress, it's probably a good idea to change your routine in some respect almost every trip to the gym, says Dr. Lefavi.

For example, if you're away on business and have allowed 45 minutes to train every other day, you could perform this workout as it reads today and then the next time you train, perform these exercises in the opposite order, starting with your ab work first. Just make sure that you always warm-up and stretch before starting, Dr. Lefavi says.

Fixes for Bad Workout Form

Whether it's at work or in the gym, when we're in a hurry, we get sloppy. That can really be a problem if you're a brain surgeon, but it's no small deal when you're heaving weights around either—unless you don't mind a torn rotator cuff or blown knee ligaments. Below are some of the most common exercise errors and how to avoid them.

- Bench press: Lifting your butt off the bench.
  Solution: Use about 20 percent less weight, keep your butt on the bench and feet flat on the floor. Don't forget to use a spotter.
- Lunges: Extending your knee over your feet while lunging.
  Solution: Step out farther and use a lighter weight. Keep your back straight.
- Barbell curls: Swinging the weight.
  Solution: Grind your elbows into your body and use less weight. Or slightly stagger your feet so that one foot— though shoulder-width apart—is 10 to 12 inches ahead of the other.
- Seated two-arm rows with tubing: Rounding your back.
  Solution: Stick out your chest, which should naturally straighten your back.

Weightless Workout

Warm-Up (4 minutes)
Walk, jump rope, or perform jumping jacks, squat thrusts, or similar activity. (Remember that a true warm-up increases your body's core temperature 1°F, so try to break a light sweat during the warm-up.)

Stretch (3 minutes)
Stretch the muscles to be trained. (While stretching, mentally prepare for the workout, focus on how you will move from one exercise to the next, and so on.)

Exercises (33 minutes)
Push-ups between chairs (three sets, 10 to 15 reps, 45 seconds between sets)

Decline push-ups (two sets, 10 to 15 reps, 45 seconds between sets)

Seated two-arm rows with tubing (three sets, 8 to 12 reps, 1 minute between sets)

Desk dips (three sets, 10 to 15 reps, 45 seconds between sets)

Biceps curls with tubing (two sets, 8 to 12 reps, 45 seconds between sets)

Upright rows with tubing (three sets, 8 to 12 reps, 1 minute between sets)

Squats (three sets, 10 to 15 reps, 1 minute between sets)

Lunges (two sets, 10 to 15 reps, 45 seconds between sets)

Crunches (three sets, 15 to 30 reps, 1 minute between sets)

Cooldown (3 minutes)
Perform any activity that uses large, major muscle groups in a rhythmical, continuous fashion, such as bicycling.

Stretch (2 minutes)

The Ultimate 60-Minute Workout

If you've carved an hour into your day for fitness, you're to be congratulated. For guys who have to watch every minute, this may be the ideal workout.

"By using this routine, you can really make large muscle mass gains with an amount of intensity and volume that I would say is optimal," says Armstrong Atlantic State University's Dr. Bob Lefavi. "What we're looking at here is the best volume while maintaining a high intensity, short rest routine in order to maximally stimulate your muscle groups."

The key difference between this program and The Ultimate 45-Minute Weight Workout is that you gain one exercise each for your chest, shoulders, and back—inclined bench presses, front lat pull-downs, and upright rows.

Inclined bench presses work the hard-to-reach upper part of your chest. Front lat pull-downs challenge your latissimus dorsi—the muscles of your back that create a V-shape—while upright rows train the front of your shoulders and your biceps.

Guys using the weightless program add desk push-ups and heel raises. Desk push-ups train your chest and triceps, while heel raises and other exercises like them help build your calves. "We get to add exercises without sacrificing sets, and that's really a plus," Dr. Lefavi says.

A word here on those one-minute rest sessions between sets. Some guys use them to

Weight Workout

Warm-Up (5 minutes)

Walk on a treadmill, ride a stationary bike, jump rope, or perform a similar activity. (Remember that a true warm-up increases your body's core temperature 1°F, so try to break a light sweat during the warm-up.)

Stretch (3 minutes)

Stretch the muscles to be trained. (While stretching, mentally prepare for the workout, focus on how you will move from one exercise to the next, and so on.)

Exercises (45 minutes, with some time allotted for weight adjustment)

Bench press (three sets, 8 to 12 reps, 1 minute between sets)

Inclined bench press (two sets, 8 to 12 reps, 1 minute between sets)

Barbell rows (three sets, 8 to 12 reps, 1 minute between sets)

Front lat pull-downs (two sets, 8 to 12 reps, 1 minute between sets)

Overhead triceps extensions (four sets, 10 to 15 reps, 45 seconds between sets)

Barbell curls (three sets, 10 to 15 reps, 45 seconds between sets)

Seated military press (two sets, 8 to 12 reps, 1 minute between sets)

Upright rows (two sets, 8 to 12 reps, 45 seconds between sets)

Squats (four sets, 8 to 12 reps, 1 minute between sets)

Stiff-legged dead lifts (three sets, 10 to 15 reps, 1 minute between sets)

Crunches (three sets, 15 to 30 reps, 1 minute between sets)

Cooldown (4 minutes)

Perform any activity that uses large, major muscle groups in a rhythmical, continuous fashion, such as bicycling.

Stretch (3 minutes)

chat up women or banter with buddies. Save that for outside the gym.

Instead, use those 60 seconds to evaluate the way that the exercise is affecting your body. Are you performing the movement correctly? Are you achieving complete contraction during the exercise? Is the weight too heavy or too light? Learning to listen to your body is a major factor in muscle growth, says Dr. Lefavi.

You might even want to consider using the brief downtime to flex those muscles. Flexing for 20 seconds and relaxing the muscle three times after you've finished training a body part may help make the muscle more defined. If you're not comfortable flexing in the gym, save it for the shower.

And since we're talking about making the most of your workout, don't forget to replenish your muscles' glycogen stores after you're done. Some good choices include fruit juice, rice, and potatoes.

What's Your Exercise Order?

Training your biceps or triceps before your chest or back is like eating dessert before your main course. Some guys don't think twice about exercise order, but research shows that training larger muscles first can lead to greater gains in strength and size in the same of time.

In one study researchers found that bench press performance dropped a whopping 75 percent when it followed triceps pushdowns and military presses. The same study found that squat performance dropped 22 percent when it was done last in a lower-body training routine. And lifting less weight over time obviously means less muscle growth.

The reason is simple. You need your triceps and biceps to perform a bench press. And working those smaller muscles first makes it harder to handle heavy weight. Ditto for doing barbell curls before barbell rows, or heel raises before squats.

Weightless ♟ Workout

Warm-Up (5 minutes)
Walk, jump rope, or perform jumping jacks, squat thrusts, or similar activity. (Remember that a true warm-up increases your body's core temperature 1°F, so try to break a light sweat during the warm-up.)

Stretch (3 minutes)
Stretch the muscles to be trained. (While stretching, mentally prepare for the workout, focus on how you will move from one exercise to the next, and so on.)

Exercises (45 minutes)
Push-ups between chairs (three sets, 10 to 15 reps, 45 seconds between sets)

Decline push-ups (two sets, 10 to 15 reps, 45 seconds between sets)

Desk push-ups (two sets, 10 to 15 reps, 45 seconds between sets)

Seated two-arm rows with tubing (three sets, 8 to 12 reps, 1 minute between sets)

Desk dips (four sets, 10 to 15 reps, 45 seconds between sets)

Biceps curls with tubing (three sets, 8 to 12 reps, 45 seconds between sets)

Upright rows with tubing (three sets, 8 to 12 reps, 1 minute between sets)

Squats (three sets, 10 to 15 reps, 1 minute between sets)

Lunges (two sets, 15 to 30 reps, 1 minute between sets)

Heel raises (three sets, 10 to 15 reps, 45 seconds between sets)

Crunches (three sets, 15 to 30 reps, 1 minute between sets)

Cooldown (4 minutes)
Perform any activity that uses large, major muscle groups in a rhythmical, continuous fashion, such as bicycling.

Stretch (3 minutes)

The Ultimate 90-Minute Workout

No question, you can get a great workout in less time. But when it comes to total body fitness, 90 minutes truly is the ultimate.

"Ninety minutes in the gym is an opportunity to get the most out of everything," says Armstrong Atlantic State University's Dr. Bob Lefavi. "Enough time to really stretch the muscle groups and enough time to train them, hitting each major muscle group with enough intensity to really take them to fatigue."

You'll note that both routines suggest up to five sets for many of the exercises. Doing five sets allows you to perform a warm-up set so that you can prepare the specific muscles that are about to be taxed. Large, thick muscles such as the quads, chest, and lats seem to respond best when your workout is preceded by a blood-pumping warm-up.

"When I say warm-up, I don't mean easy. I mean lighter weight. Fifteen to 20 reps with a lighter weight gets the blood flowing to the muscle group, preparing it to go a little harder and a little longer with that movement," Dr. Lefavi says.

For the warm-up set, Dr. Lefavi suggests using weights that represent 40 to 70 percent of what you normally use. Of course, for the weightless workout, you can't use a lighter weight for the warm-up. But you can add more

Weight Workout

Warm-Up (6 minutes)
Walk, jump rope, or perform jumping jacks, squat thrusts, or similar activity. (Remember that a true warm-up increases your body's core temperature 1°F, so try to break a light sweat during the warm-up.)

Stretch (4 minutes)
Stretch the muscles to be trained. (While stretching, mentally prepare for the workout, focus on how you will move from one exercise to the next, and so on.)

Exercises (70 minutes, with some time allotted for weight adjustment)

Bench press (five sets, 8 to 12 reps, 90 seconds between sets; first set as warm-up set)

Inclined bench press (four sets, 8 to 12 reps, 75 seconds between sets)

Barbell rows (five sets, 8 to 12 reps, 90 seconds between sets; first set as a warm-up set)

Front lat pull-downs (four sets, 8 to 12 reps, 75 seconds between sets)

Overhead triceps extensions (five sets, 10 to 15 reps, 45 seconds between sets; first set as warm-up set)

Barbell curls (four sets, 10 to 15 reps, 45 seconds between sets)

Seated military press (four sets, 8 to 12 reps, 1 minute between sets)

Upright rows (three sets, 8 to 12 reps, 1 minute between sets)

Squats (five sets, 8 to 12 reps, 90 seconds between sets; first set as warm-up set)

Stiff-legged dead lifts (four sets, 10 to 15 reps, 1 minute between sets)

Crunches (five sets, 15 to 30 reps, 1 minute between sets)

Cooldown (6 minutes)
Perform any activity that uses large, major muscle groups in a rhythmical, continuous fashion, such as bicycling.

Stretch (4 minutes)

stretching through the motion you're about to do and make sure that the first set is done slowly, Dr. Lefavi says.

Just don't go *too* long. Working out for much more than 90 minutes can upset the delicate balance of hormones—such as testosterone and cortisol—thereby inhibiting muscle growth. "To maximize testosterone levels, the body wants training sessions that are hard and brief. Once it starts to look like you're going to go hard for too long a time . . . that's when the body says, this isn't a good stress, it's a bad stress. And that's when stress hormones jump and testosterone levels drop," he says.

Don't be surprised if, after performing this many exercises and sets, you're extremely sore. Just remember: Unlike any sharp pain you might feel during your workout—which should always make you stop what you're doing and seek professional help—some muscle soreness hours after your workout is normal, Dr. Lefavi says.

"When you put a muscle in a stress that it's not accustomed to, you create microscopic tears in the muscle fibers that attract water, which, in turn, causes swelling, pressure on nerve receptors, and, eventually, pain—or at least that's one theory," Dr. Lefavi says.

In fact, it's probably best not to train that particular muscle again until it's no longer sore to the touch—usually 48 to 72 hours later, says Dr. Lefavi.

"Your muscle is slowly putting back more protein to rebuild. Now if you don't let that repair go on long enough and you short-circuit it by training too hard too soon, you will—over time—cause overtraining."

And now for perhaps the best part of your workout: Rest. It's during the rest stage that your muscles repair themselves, growing bigger and stronger. Try to get between seven and eight hours of shut-eye a night if you work out hard and often.

Weightless Workout

Warm-Up (6 minutes)

Walk, jump rope, or perform jumping jacks, squat thrusts, or similar activity. (Remember that a true warm-up increases your body's core temperature 1°F, so try to break a light sweat during the warm-up.)

Stretch (4 minutes)

Stretch the muscles to be trained. (While stretching, mentally prepare for the workout, focus on how you will move from one exercise to the next, and so on.)

Exercises (70 minutes)

Push-ups between chairs (five sets, 10 to 15 reps, 1 minute between sets)

Decline push-ups (four sets, 10 to 15 reps, 45 seconds between sets)

Desk push-ups (two sets, 10 to 15 reps, 45 seconds between sets)

Seated two-arm rows with tubing (five sets, 8 to 12 reps, 1 minute between sets)

Desk dips (five sets, 10 to 15 reps, 1 minute between sets)

Biceps curls with tubing (five sets, 8 to 12 reps, 45 seconds between sets)

Upright rows with tubing (five sets, 8 to 12 reps, 1 minute between sets)

Squats (five sets, 10 to 15 reps, 1 minute between sets)

Lunges (four sets, 10 to 15 reps, 45 seconds between sets)

Heel raises (three sets, 10 to 15 reps, 45 seconds between sets)

Crunches (five sets, 15 to 30 reps, 1 minute between sets)

Cooldown (6 minutes)

Perform any activity that uses large, major muscle groups in a rhythmical, continuous fashion, such as bicycling.

Stretch (4 minutes)

Basketball

Courting a Better Workout

Chances are that you fall short of the average NBA player . . . in more than just height. The typical pro hoopster earns nearly $1.9 million per year, higher than any other team sport. And what does he have to do to get all that dough? Play the game you wish you had more time to play. Your schedule is filled with meetings, lunches, and conference calls. His schedule is filled with . . . games.

Years ago, you gave up any dreams of playing in the NBA. Or the CBA. Or even the YMCA league. And unless you hit the lottery, odds are that you aren't going to be quitting your nine-to-five job anytime soon to perfect your three-pointer. So your only real choice is to make the most of the time you do manage to spend on the court.

Hoops—There It Is

"Unlike professionals, most regular guys play basketball only occasionally—like on Saturday mornings," says Ron Culp, president of the NBA Trainers Association and team trainer for the Miami Heat and the 1996 U.S. Olympic Dream Team. "And that's why they pay the price on Sunday and take about a week to recover."

You may not have time to play hoops more than one or two times a week, but there are steps that you can take—without getting called for walking—to turn up the intensity and to rebound quickly. Here are some tips to employ before the next tip-off.

Play full court. "Most pickup games are played half-court, but if you really want a killer workout, make it full

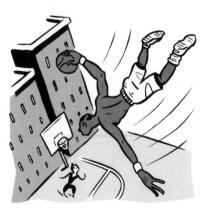

court," suggests Tom LaGarde, former center with the 1979 NBA champion Seattle Supersonics and a member of the gold medal–winning 1976 U.S. Olympic basketball team.

"One of the hardest things you can do in basketball is play one-on-one full court, but even a three-on-three full-court game will kick your butt and give you an incredible workout in a small amount of time," says LaGarde. "Anything that makes you run up and down the court continuously will get you in great shape fast."

Be like Mike. Sure, Michael Jordan took the art of scoring to new heights. But what *really* makes him the greatest ever is his ferocious defense. Now, if Jordan is willing to play D, what's your excuse? "Many recreational players, when they don't have the ball, tend to stand around with their hands on their hips, *waiting* for the ball," LaGarde says.

"But if you only have an hour or so and want to get the best workout you can, keep moving all the time in order to keep your heart rate up," says LaGarde. "Playing defense is a great way to keep moving, but even on offense, always move so that the guy playing defense on you always has to move."

Beat the clock. The NBA uses a 24-second shot clock to keep the game moving. College players have 45 seconds to get a shot off. So if you're tired of wasting too much time on the court standing around while some clown puts on a dribbling exhibition, try using a game clock. Set a time limit—24, 30, or 45 seconds—to put up a shot or else the ball goes to the other side.

Do laps before layups. Actually, if you want to *survive* that full-court game and ferocious defense, Culp suggests that you run around the perimeter of the court three or four times before hitting the hardwood. "Basketball is an anaerobic sport, and the only way to get the quick energy you need for a better workout and a better game is to run," he says. "You need to warm up your muscles before actually playing in order to prevent injuries and increase your endurance."

Not into laps? "Try walking to the gym instead of riding," suggests Culp. "Or if you're playing on your lunch hour, walk down the stairs instead of taking the elevator." Of course, he also recommends a regular road workout to boost both anaerobic and aerobic endurance. "If you want to play ball—even for an hour—play on Monday, Wednesday, and Friday and run sprints on Tuesday, Thursday, and Saturday. The single best thing you can do to get more from your basketball workout is to run."

Stretch. If you only have an hour or so to play, chances are that you don't want to spend 10 minutes of it stretching. Big mistake.

"As you age, the first thing to go is flexibility, which is why so many guys have sore backs and knees after playing," Culp says. "I can't stress enough how important it is to stretch before and after playing. By stretching, you not only improve your flexibility so that you're less likely to get injured but also improve your workout because your body will be able to handle the game." He suggests paying particular attention to your lower back, hamstrings, groin, Achilles tendons, and Achilles' heels with a series of stretches to improve range of motion.

Make like Carl Lewis. If you want to increase your vertical leap and build stronger legs, practice this move, suggests Mike Brungardt, strength and conditioning coach for the NBA's San Antonio Spurs and co-author of *The Complete Book of Butt and Legs*. Just stand with your knees slightly bent and arms relaxed at your sides, and then jump forward, as if you were doing a broad jump.

Cross-Training ⚡ Tip

Play enough basketball and one of two things will likely happen to the average guy. You'll wind up either on a Wheaties box or at an orthopedic surgeon's office.

"I stopped playing because of my knees, and as most players know, basketball is very demanding on the knees," says Tom LaGarde, formerly of the Seattle Supersonics. "So that leaves you in a catch-22 situation: You can either stay off the court so that your knees don't hurt from playing, but then you don't get the aerobic conditioning you need for the game, or play and have your knees hurt, in which case you can't play for too long and again you don't get the aerobic conditioning you need."

But LaGarde suggests a third option that saves both your knees and your game: in-line skating. "Skating is a great cross-trainer for just about any sport, but it's really great for basketball."

So great, in fact, that he started the National In-Line Basketball League (NIBBL), which has teams in many U.S. and Canadian cities. Guys play a regular game of basketball while wearing in-line skates, saving their knees and improving their "regular" game.

"In-line skating helps improve basketball in three ways," says LaGarde. "It won't hurt your knees. It gives you better balance for all sports, including basketball. And it forces you to really concentrate on shot making, which translates to being a better shooter in basketball." For more information on the NIBBL, call (212) 539-1132.

But as you land—with knees bent to absorb the shock—jump again, this time raising your arms over your head to lift you higher. Make the second jump as quickly as possible to increase speed and strength. Do 8 to 10 repetitions.

Bicycling

Getting in Gear

Cycling may be a fast way to get where you're going. But it can be darn slow in taking you where you want to go.

"Unfortunately, outdoor cycling doesn't lend itself to getting a quick *and* effective workout, because it takes more time than running and other sports," says Chris Kostman, an elite cyclist who pedaled his way from San Francisco to Washington, D.C., in just 10 days and who is on the executive board of the Ultra Marathon Cycling Association in Canyon, Texas, a group that sanctions cycling races totaling more than 300 miles per day. "It's really hard to get a whole lot done in just 45 minutes or an hour a day."

"The advantage of a bicycle for an athlete," adds Len Pettyjohn, Ph.D., a coach and trainer in Denver who used to run the Coors Light Cycling Team, "is that it's nonload-bearing, so you don't get the problems with your hips and ankles like you do in other sports. But that's also its disadvantage. Because a bike is so efficient, you have to work really hard to get a good workout—especially if you don't have a lot of time."

On a Roll

Just to give you an idea of what you're up against, the average guy who weighs 176 pounds burns 160 calories in 20 minutes of cycling. That's roughly the same number he would burn if he spent the same amount of time playing Frisbee or badminton.

But there are ways to gain added benefits from cycling even over shorter

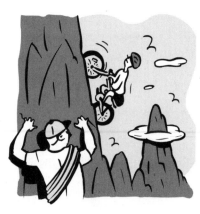

periods of time. And it's especially useful for overweight and out-of-shape men, because the bike, rather than their joints, supports the extra poundage. So saddle up and get ready to ride.

Assume the position. "To get the best workout, you have to be positioned on the bike correctly," says John Howard, a three-time Olympic cyclist from Encinitas, California, and one of the most respected technicians in the sport. "You need the right leg extension—with knees bent slightly at a 30- to 35-degree angle at the bottom dead-center, or six o'clock, position. Too much knee bend will cause you to ride incorrectly and fatigue you too early. On the downstroke (when your foot is closest to the ground), your toe should drop to a six o'clock position, so that your toes are pointed to the ground. And your back should be comfortably flat on about a 45-degree angle."

Be a mountain man. "If you go off on a mountain bike and tackle some hilly terrain, you have no choice but to get a great workout, even if it's only for an hour," says Dan Buettner of Minneapolis, who holds three world records in distance cycling—for riding across the Soviet Union, across Africa, and from Alaska to South America. "Besides the hills, the rough terrain creates more resistance, so you have to work harder. And it's a lot more exciting than the monotony of following the yellow lines of a road."

Mountain biking is especially good for guys who want to cycle after work. "Rush hour is the worst time to ride because of the number of vehicles and the level of carbon monoxide," Dr. Pettyjohn explains. "But with mountain biking, you don't have to worry about cars or pollution."

Keep tabs on your ticker. The key to a more intense cycling workout is to push your heart rate up. "Almost all good athletes, and I would suggest many weekend athletes as well, should get a heart rate monitor so that they can get up to their target heart range," states Dr. Pettyjohn.

To determine your maximum heart rate, take your age minus 20 and multiply that by 0.67. Then subtract that number from 200. That means a 30-year-old man would have a maximum heart rate of 193 (rounded off) beats per minute. Most experts suggest a 5- to 10-minute warm-up riding at a "walking pace," then spending the majority of your cycling time pedaling so that your heart rate is between 70 and 90 percent of your maximum rate—in this case, anywhere from 135 to 174 (rounded off) beats per minute. Then end your workout with a 5- to 10-minute cooldown by riding slowly, again at a walking pace.

Start packing. "When I prepare for a race, I usually load panniers on my bike; they're like saddlebags," Buettner says. "The extra weight can give you a better workout than riding without them."

Practice indoors. "The biggest problem in not getting a good workout for busy guys is that they spend too much time coasting when riding outdoors because of traffic and terrain—not to mention the time you spend changing flat tires," Kostman says. "So if you have a limited time to go cycling, I recommend riding on a stationary bike."

Kostman teaches classes in spinning, in which cyclists ride on a special stationary bike that has a fixed gear similar to a track bicycle. "You can't coast in spinning, so you're always pedaling. The classes I teach are only 45 minutes long, but you get a workout that's probably three times better than spending the same amount of time riding on the road outdoors."

If there are no spinning classes at a health club near you and you want to use your road bike indoors, he recommends using rollers rather than indoor trainers. "Rollers consist of three drums connected with a rubber band. One drum is under your front wheel, and two

Cross-Training Tip

Being able to contort your body like a pretzel may not keep you from winding up like one after a bad spill, but yoga and similar disciplines can better prepare cyclists for all that the road offers.

"Like any other activity, cycling overemphasizes certain muscles and de-emphasizes others," says Chris Kostman of the Ultra Marathon Cycling Association. "And what happens in cycling is that you tend to get really tight hamstrings and glute muscles as well as those in your back. So you need to do something that balances the fact that you are overdoing those muscles, because having a wider range of motion is really critical for using your body efficiently."

That's why he recommends yoga or a similar discipline to increase range of motion. "Flexibility is something that's very often overlooked in cycling, but it's so important," he says. "If all you're doing is riding a bike and your legs are only moving in a circle, then you may have trouble with lateral movement or even lifting your legs for things like hiking. But yoga can help you increase that range of motion."

are under your rear wheel. With a Windtrainer, you lock your rear wheel into a stand, and there's a device that your back wheel pedals against to create resistance."

The difference is that, with rollers, you must balance yourself, so besides getting a good cardiovascular workout, you foster a smooth pedaling style and finesse. "With rollers, if you're not smooth, you fall off," says Kostman. "But Windtrainers can foster sloppy riding style, because your bike is locked in place."

Rollers will set you back between $300 and $500, while indoor trainers generally cost between $150 and $300.

Golf

Be Game for a Better Workout

That classic battle between the tortoise and hare taught a valuable lesson—and not only to bookies: Slow and steady wins the race, despite the point spread.

That also applies to longevity. While there's no arguing that any regular exercise can prolong your life, research now shows that too much of a good thing may be counter-productive. Translation: Lower-intensity, longer-duration activities may be a better bet for the George Burns route than shorter periods of intense exercise.

Experts studying this area of sports science are beginning to see a surprising number of ultra athletes and marathon runners who are among the most fit in the world but who are still coming down with medical problems, including cancer and heart disease. "That's because extremely high levels of exercise can weaken the immune system, making you more susceptible to certain diseases," says Kenneth Cooper, M.D., president and founder of the Cooper Aerobics Center in Dallas and the so-called Father of Aerobics.

But guess who's living long enough to enjoy their retirement on the links?

Stay on the Right Course

Golf has long had a reputation for providing opportunities for flexing your corporate muscle but not much else. Sure, you have to be reasonably fit to avoid injury and smack the ball 300 yards, but let's face it—a lot of golfers don't exactly look like Adonis.

But with the new

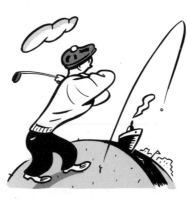

emphasis on longer periods of moderate exercise, playing golf offers some very real potential health benefits.

The problem is that it takes about 4½ hours to complete those 18 holes. And most golfers are interested in playing better, not faster. In fact, the sport's leisurely pace is one of its most appealing traits. So the question becomes not how to slash the amount of time you spend on the course but how to gain the maximum health and fitness benefits while you're out there. We're glad you asked.

Don't go à la cart. Considering that you only spend a total of about two minutes actually hitting the ball in that 4½-hour round, common sense dictates that you'll get a better workout walking the course—burning a minimum of 270 calories an hour and giving your heart a good aerobic workout, says Greg Johnson, director of the golf program at Health-South Rehabilitation Corporation in Atlanta and athletic trainer on the Professional Golfers' Association tour.

One other advantage to walking the course is that you'll be less likely to hurt your back, the most common golf injury, says Johnson. "There's a lot of evidence that suggests that it's riding in a cart that's the cause of many golf-related back injuries," Johnson says. "The constant vibrations of riding in a cart put too much stress and strain on your back, similar to what occurs when you're driving a truck."

Give soreness the cold shoulder. Carrying a bag of clubs can turn your shoulders into mush. "What I recommend is that on holes 1, 3, 5, 7, and so on, you carry your golf bag on one shoulder, and that on the even-numbered holes, you carry it on the other side," Johnson says. "Most people tend to carry their bag on one shoulder, which not only leaves them sore but also results in their dropping one shoulder—and not playing as well as they could. Or buy a universal strap (about $15) that allows you to carry your clubs in the middle of your back.

"And if you're pulling your clubs with a small cart, switch around: Push the cart on some holes and pull it on alternating holes. And use both your right and left hands so that you more evenly distribute the load to both sides of your body, reducing the risk of strain."

Stretch at each hole. After golf carts, most injuries—and scores that resemble a bowling game—come from hitting the links immediately after the course parking lot, says Johnson. If you start swinging without stretching first, your muscles are cold, Johnson warns. As a result, your game will be, too. But don't assume that a couple of quick stretches before the first tee are sufficient. "I advise that whenever you're waiting for someone else to shoot, stretch."

Golf legend Gary Player likes to lay a club across the back of his shoulders, grab both ends with his hands, and slowly twist from side to side. Other essential stretches you can do between holes include a back extension, where you place your hands on your hips and lean backward; shoulder stretches, where you clasp your hands behind your back and move your arms upward; bending side to side with your arms grasped overhead; and stretching your hamstrings, says Johnson.

Give your game a lift. One way to get through a round of golf faster is to simply hit the ball farther each time. And weight lifting can help you do that.

A study conducted at the PGA National Resort and Spa in Palm Beach Gardens, Florida, followed golfers who embarked on a fitness program using exercise machines and free weights. At the end of 12 weeks, 85 percent of the exercisers increased the distance that they could hit the ball by 15 yards, on average.

Cross-Training Tip

As one of America's premier milers, Steve Scott has run up all kinds of records: member of three U.S. Olympic track teams; 136 sub-four-minute miles, including the American record; and oh, yeah, the former Guinness world record for playing the fastest round of golf. The time: 29 minutes, 30 seconds for 18 holes. The score: 95—about five strokes higher than his regular game.

"I got interested in speed golf after doing it with my friends a couple of times, but it's definitely helped my running," says Scott, of San Diego. "I get a great workout without realizing that I'm getting one, because I'm so busy thinking about my last shot or my next shot that I don't have time to think about how tired I am from running the course full blast."

With speed golf, you carry one ball and up to three clubs (Scott prefers a three iron, wedge, and putter). Wearing running shoes and shorts, you run the course all out between shots. The fastest time wins.

"Theoretically, it's probably not a great idea for your golf game, because you're not hitting the ball properly because you're so rushed," says Scott, who set the speed golf record in 1979 and held it for eight years. "But it forces you to hit the ball straight. If you slice or hook, you'll be running a lot longer to retrieve your ball."

If you want to try it, Scott offers the following advice. "Go early: If you're not first on the course, forget it. Pack lightly: I used only a three iron when I got the world record. And don't run too hard going up hills, or else you'll tire yourself out."

In-Line Skating

It's the Wheel Thing

Remember *Kansas City Bomber*, the 1972 epic film in which a skimpily clad Raquel Welch played a roller-derby diva who exchanged elbows and bad dialogue with other foxy four-wheelers? The movie may have lived up to its title at the box office, but it proved one thing: Roller skating can certainly get your heart rate going. Just ask the guys watching it.

Today, with more scientific data to rely on, researchers have come to the same conclusion as those testosterone-fueled film buffs. Skating, even when it doesn't involve Raquel, can get the pulse rate up as much as running and burns even more calories, says Joel Rappelfeld, founder of Roll America In-Line Skate School in New York City, a professional in-line skater, and author of *The Complete Blader*, considered by some to be the bible of the sport. Rappelfeld, who also has done a video, *Get Started in Blading*, says that in-line skating can torch up to 700 calories in one hour, making it one of the most time-productive workouts there is.

"Many people don't realize just how great of a workout you can get from in-line skating," says Rappelfeld. "It gives you a fabulous aerobic workout and works all the major muscle groups, particularly in the lower body."

Skating through Life

Of course, few guys have the time for the intense daily workouts practiced by Rappelfeld, who has taught Diana Ross, Howard Stern's sidekick Robin Quivers, and

other celebrities how to street-skate at Roll America. So what can we do to get the most from our in-line skating?

Show variety. The best way to get the most out of your in-line skating is to vary your routine. "Too many people get out there and just glide around," Rappelfeld says. "But in order to get good, you need to mix things up in your workout. Once you're comfortable on your in-line skates, start with long, low strides and practice that for about five minutes, and then sprint for one to two minutes. By adding intensity, you'll get the most workout in the shortest amount of time."

Get in line. "One of the biggest mistakes that most in-line skaters make is with their form," Rappelfeld says. "They stand too straight and keep their knees locked, like Frankenstein. Instead, your skating position should be like a skier, with your nose, knees, and toes in alignment with each other."

In proper position, you're leaning forward from the waist and bent at the knees, so a straight, slightly diagonal line could be drawn hitting the tip of your nose, your knees, and your toes. Besides putting more stress on your joints, an incorrect skating position makes it easier to fall, and you have to skate harder to keep moving. "Knees should be flexed at all times, to act as shock absorbers," Rappelfeld says. To help lower your position, try it with your elbows on your knees, which really gives your legs a good workout, lengthens your stride, and helps improve your form.

Do it daily. Maybe you don't have four hours a day to devote to in-line skating, like Ryan Jacklone, the 1995 Aggressive Skating Association world champion from New York City. "But to be a better skater, you have to make it part of your daily ritual—even if it's only for a few minutes," Jacklone says. "That may mean strapping on your in-lines to go to the corner to buy the newspaper or a quart of milk. But the people who make the most of their time skating are those who make time for skating every day, even if it's only for five minutes."

Use those arms. Swinging your arms front to back keeps you in better balance and is advised when you're sprinting, according to Rappelfeld.

He suggests skating with arms behind your back, like a speed ice skater. "Start with one arm behind your back, and when you're comfortable in that position, put the other arm behind your back. With both arms behind you, you're working the lower body more and strengthening your leg muscles more quickly." If you feel that you are out of balance with two arms behind your back, practice with just one arm behind you (alternating left and right every once in a while to get used to both) until you are comfortable. Eventually, you will be able to skate with both arms behind you.

Get into all-wheel drive. The correct way to push off is with all your wheels. "Most people push off on their toes, so their stroke ends with their heel up, which can result in falling," says Rappelfeld. "So make sure that you stroke out to the side using all your wheels and recover letting your foot back in close to the other foot."

In-line on an incline. Studies show that running or cycling gives you a better aerobic workout than in-line skating does. The reason is that, with in-line skating, you're gliding—in other words, resting—between strokes. But here's a simple way to ratchet up the intensity— provided you're not a flatlander. Find a long, gradual incline and repeatedly skate up it, then rest by walking back down the hill. In-line

Cross-Training ⚡ Tip

For serious skaters like Roll America In-Line Skate School's Joel Rappelfeld, the man who teaches many of New York's rich and famous how to deal with those wheels, time isn't always the biggest obstacle.

Mother Nature is.

"Basically, in-line skating means that you're at the mercy of the weather," he says. "You can't do it when it rains or snows." But even when the weather is bad, you still can condition yourself to be hell on wheels.

"I complement my skating with bicycling and using a horizontal slide board. With bicycling, you use similar muscles to those used in skating, and it definitely has increased my endurance. And whenever the weather is bad, I pull out the horizontal slide board and use it in my home."

A horizontal slide board is a sheet of plastic that can be used to simulate the skating motion. They are available at some sporting goods shops for under $100. "With a slide board, you do the same routine you would use skating: long, smooth, and easy strokes followed by shorter, more intense, sprinting-type motions," Rappelfeld says.

skating uphill provides an aerobic workout that you would only get at dangerously high speeds on flat ground.

Mix it up. For an innovative full-body workout, Rappelfeld suggests combining skating with other simple exercises. For instance, skate for 10 minutes, then stop and do some crunches. Skate for 10 minutes more, then hit the ground for some push-ups. And since each skate weighs three to five pounds, you can even use them for leg lifts.

Running

Racing the Clock

You say that you don't have time to run? Consider Clarence DeMar.

From the age of 16, DeMar worked hard. He paid for his schooling by pitching hay, cutting corn, and performing other farm chores. He also worked beating rugs and in print shops. When he turned 21, he left the University of Vermont to work in a print shop to support his mother and the rest of his family.

Throughout his adult life, DeMar worked as a compositor in various print shops around Boston while attending night school to earn an associate's degree from Harvard University and a master's degree from Boston University.

Oh, and in his spare time he managed to squeeze in enough running to win seven Boston Marathons between 1911 and 1930—a truly remarkable record. Usually, DeMar trained for his races by running to and from work, carrying a dry shirt with him.

Now, you were saying?

Timely Treks

DeMar once said of his sport: "Running has several advantages as a pastime. It is economical in cost of equipment and in the space required, and the time is optimal. It is not dangerous to life or limb, and it usually improves health."

Indeed. Although running is among the most time-efficient exercises you'll find—you burn about 100 calories per mile, which takes most male

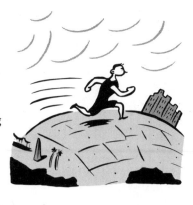

recreational runners anywhere from 8 to 10 minutes—DeMar is one of the few working stiffs who succeeded in making time for a world-class workout.

"If you want to achieve a high level of fitness, the rules are well-established: You drive the heart into the target heart zone (a range that's between 70 and 90 percent of the maximum number of beats your heart can produce) and keep it there for 20 to 30 continuous minutes, and you do this several times a week," says Bryant Stamford, Ph.D., director of the Health Promotion and Wellness Center at the University of Louisville and author of *Fitness without Exercise.* "The question is, does everyone in America have the time to do this? The answer is 'No.'"

So here's how to get the most from running when you're racing the clock.

Take a hint—and sprint. Most casual runners with limited time make the same mistake: They hit the road at a comfortable pace and go for quantity over quality.

"If you want to make the most of your workout with a limited amount of time, you need to pick up the intensity. Instead of running three to five miles at the same pace each time, you need to run a lot of short, fast intervals—like run for 40 seconds really hard and then jog or even walk for a minute one or two times a week," says Steve Spence, a world-class marathoner from Chambersburg, Pennsylvania, who won a bronze medal in the 1991 World Championships and was a member of the 1992 U.S. Olympic team. "Your overall distance might be a little less this way, but you'll get a better workout in the time that you spend."

One of America's premier milers, Steve Scott, suggests doing these intervals at a nearby high school track. "Run the straightaways at a sprintlike pace and ease up on the curves—and you'll get a great workout in a limited time," he recommends.

If there's no track nearby, Spence suggests gauging your intervals by counting the number of telephone poles as you're running on the street. "You sprint for two or three poles, and then jog or walk for one or two," Spence says.

Choose the right surface. And that's *not* asphalt. "My advice is to try to run on a dirt track or find someplace that's grassy or has another soft surface," Scott says. "You really pound yourself too much running on asphalt." The problem—especially for guys with limited time—is that running on hard surfaces increases your risk of injuries, joint pain, and shinsplints. Besides, the pain of running on a hard surface tends to slow your pace, progress, and desire, Scott warns.

Take the scenic route. You think you're busy? Try running a country. "President Clinton has a very busy schedule, but he still manages to run several miles a time, several days a week, at an eight-minute-per-mile pace," says Mary Ann Hill, director of communications for the President's Council on Physical Fitness and Sports in Washington, D.C. "While the route he runs is chosen largely with security in mind, he often runs in areas like parks because of the scenery and because it is less disruptive to traffic."

Even if you don't have a bunch of Secret Service agents to absorb the impact of an oncoming two-ton Chevy, common sense dictates that if you have to constantly dodge traffic or other distractions, you'll probably dodge running.

"If the only time you can run is after work and it's too dark and you don't want to

---

Cross-Training ⚡Tip

Even though Olympic marathoner Steve Spence runs more often than Bob Dole and complements his roadwork with weights and nightly calisthenics, some of his best leg strengthening comes from an unlikely source: shooting hoops.

"I don't play in games, because there's too much of a risk of getting injured coming down on someone's ankle. But just shooting around and playing games like Horse is really good for my running," he says. "With running, all your muscles are used to going forward, but there's not a lot of side-to-side motion.

"But playing basketball is a great way to strengthen the lower legs because of all the lateral movement. It's a great warm-up for me, because with all the stopping and turning, it helps loosen my leg muscles before a run. I recommend basketball for anyone who runs."

---

risk going on the road, try running in a mall parking lot," advises Spence. "They tend to be better lit and less crowded than streets. What I do during bad weather or at night is go to a parking lot—usually a school—and run a three- or four-minute loop 10 times or so."

Climb every mountain. "Too many people always go on a flat route, but an excellent way to get the most from running, especially with limited time, is to include hills in your workout," Spence says.

"My advice is to sprint up a hill for about 30 seconds and jog down. But be sure that the hills aren't too steep—ideally a 4 or 5 percent grade. Anything more and it may be too much." And if you're running indoors on a treadmill, be sure to include inclines every few minutes.

Skiing

Path to Fitness Is All Downhill

You've spent several hours Friday night driving through snow and ice on treacherous two-lane mountain roads to reach the ski lodge. Now, all you can think about is how to spend every possible minute of the next 48 hours on the slopes.

"The object of skiing is not to get a great workout in the least amount of time but to enjoy a full day on the mountain and let the workout be a side benefit," says Jeff Hamilton, who holds the world record for speed skiing, at 150 miles per hour.

Because of the nature of the sport, there won't be many occasions when you'll find yourself trying to get the absolute most out of 20 minutes of skiing. But for most of us, skiing isn't a sport that we can do every day. If you have the time and money, you're lucky to get in semi-regular weekend trips four or five months out of the year.

So the issues become how to stay in shape year-round so that you can enjoy your favorite sport and how to make the most of the precious time you are able to spend on the slopes.

"Too many people underestimate the skills and training needed in skiing," says Bob Barnes, director of the Skier Improvement Center at Winter Park Ski Area in Winter Park, Colorado, and a member of the U.S. Ski Instructors National Team. "They're not adequately prepared, and as a result, they get injured."

Do they ever. There were more than 126,000 skiing

injuries in 1995 that required emergency-room treatment.

Shushing for Success

Skiing requires strength, power, and quickness, so most experts recommend hitting the weights before the slopes. And since it also requires agility and flexibility, stretching is very important, says Barnes. And when you're paying more than $30 for an afternoon on the slopes, you want to make sure that you're getting your money's worth, so endurance-building activities such as running and cycling are in order.

While you're on the slopes, here's how to keep your skiing workouts from going downhill and get the most from every minute on the mountain.

Practice those turns. "One of the best ways to get your heart rate up while skiing for a better workout, as well as to improve your skiing style, is to do a lot of short-radius turning—changing direction every 10 feet or so," says Barnes. "Making a lot of short turns takes more effort than doing long cruising turns, and you have to work your muscles harder."

If you're going to throw in a lot of turns, though, you need to know the proper form. Although it appears that most skiers are standing squarely on both feet, this is an

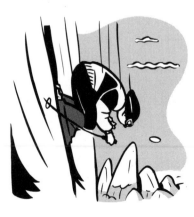

illusion. Ninety-five percent of your weight should be on the ski that's on the outside of the turn. (Weight on the right ski to turn left; weight on the left ski to turn right.) Between turns, transfer your weight onto the other ski. Now you're ready to turn in the other direction.

Go nonstop. Too many guys take frequent breaks during longer runs, but to get the best workout, Barnes suggests tackling the entire run nonstop. "For real efficiency, the fitness-minded skier shouldn't stop—from the top of the mountain to the bottom in one continuous run." This may work your muscles harder, but it's energy well-spent. "You'll always get a better workout if you don't stop, and it's a great way to keep your heart rate up," he says.

Look for "bad" conditions. Fresh powder may be a skier's dream, but for a better workout, look for wetter conditions. "While skiing in powder is strenuous and gives you a good workout because it's harder to keep your balance, when snow is wet, it's even harder to ski in, so you'll get a more strenuous workout," he says. "Icy snow, which occurs after wet snow freezes, is also good for getting a good workout and improving your performance."

Keep your balance. If you want to stay on your skis all afternoon, it helps to be in a comfortable, balanced position. "Probably the biggest mistake skiers make is that they lean back too much, which burns their thighs and can make them end their skiing day too early," Hamilton says.

By staying balanced in a neutral position, there's less effort placed on your thighs, and you'll be able to ski for hours longer. "What you need to do is bend your knees and make a conscious effort to feel your shins hitting the top of your ski boots without bending too much at the waist," Hamilton says.

Do squat. It's become your winter ritual: You spend the weekend skiing and Monday nursing sore muscles. The aches go away in a few days, but they return after your next trip to the slopes. Why? Because you're only using those leg muscles once a week, says Steve Johnson, Ph.D., professor of sports science at the University of Utah in Salt Lake

Cross-Training Tip

Even when there's no snow on the mountain, you can still head there to improve your skiing skills. Just make sure you bring a bike.

"One of the best things you can do to become a better skier is to ride a mountain bike in the off-season," says Bob Barnes of the Skier Improvement Center at Winter Park Ski Area. "Mountain biking is the perfect cross-training activity because you're traveling over variables in terrain while trying to maintain control, just as in skiing. It's also great because it works the same leg muscles as skiing and requires good balance that you need to be a good skier."

"Road biking is good for the big burn," adds speed skiing world-record holder Jeff Hamilton, "but skiing is more of a sprinting activity—and riding a mountain bike in varied terrain is perfect for simulating the sprint/rest cycles of skiing."

City and director of sports science for U.S. Skiing in Park City, Utah.

To sidestep postskiing soreness, you have to exercise your "skiing muscles" between trips. Dr. Johnson recommends doing balance squats on Tuesday and Thursday. They strengthen the thigh and calf muscles by mimicking the bent-knee crouch you're in while skiing.

Here's how to do them. Stand 8 to 10 inches in front of a chair, facing away from it. Bend your left knee to rest your left foot on the edge of the chair. Keeping your back straight and arms at your sides, slowly squat. Stop before your right thigh becomes parallel with the floor. Push yourself back up until your right leg is straight. Do 12 to 15 repetitions, then repeat the exercise to work your left leg.

Swimming

Different Strokes for Busy Folks

Working a swim into your busy workday isn't easy. But it can be done.

Just look at former President John Quincy Adams. On second thought, you'd better not look.

It seems that Adams swam across the Potomac River almost every morning with his steward, Antoine Guista. Both of them were stark naked. The mere thought of any of our recent presidents reenacting Adams's morning ritual is too horrific to even contemplate. But if the chief executive of the most powerful nation on earth can find time for a swim, maybe—just maybe—you can, too.

But, please, bring your swimsuit.

Diving In

Swimming has a lot going for it. It's a safe, effective way to boost strength and aerobic capacity without pounding your joints and other body parts the way other sports do. And a typical 180-pound guy can burn 630 calories in an hour doing a slow crawl—about the same he would lose tackling hilly terrain on a gnat-infested hike or risking frostbite going cross-country skiing.

But let's face it, time-efficient it ain't. There's the drive to the pool, changing into your suit, and maybe even the required shower before hitting the pool. As if that wasn't enough to drown your enthusiasm, most recreational swimmers spend what little time they can in the water doing a workout that's all wet.

"Most recreational swimmers go to a pool and just do

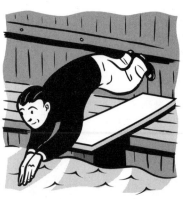

the same thing—swim laps in their favorite stroke," says "Spanky" Stephens, head athletic trainer at the University of Texas in Austin. "And that's why they never really improve or get the most from their swimming workouts."

If you want to get more out of your time in the pool, here's what Stephens and other experts recommend.

Put a cap on laps. "If you want to get the best workout in a short time period, probably the worst thing that you can do is to just swim laps at a comfortable pace," says Drury Gallagher, a New York City business executive who holds 10 world "Masters" swimming records and who, in 1983, set the one-time world record for swimming around Manhattan Island. "To improve your cardiovascular training and overall swimming, you need interval training—mixing up your routine and really going hard at 70 to 85 percent of your maximum speed," says Gallagher. "Push your pulse rate up with the fast pace, then slow down on the rest period."

So instead of swimming, say, 40 laps at the same pace, he recommends breaking it up into 10 four-lap or 20 two-lap swims, with a rest break of 10 to 20 seconds. Start slowly, but with each drill, try to increase the speed. "And mix up your routine—sometimes I just kick for one lap and swim one lap, with a 10- to 20-second rest in between," says Gallagher, considered by many to be the best American swimmer over the age of 50. "Or I'll swim one set using a pull buoy." Besides improving your swimming, it helps reduce the boredom.

Change your stroke. To be a better swimmer, practice your worst strokes. "I see a lot of guys sticking with their best stroke, usually the crawl," Stephens says. "But when you vary your strokes—do some breaststroke, some butterfly, some backstroke—you'll work muscles that you may normally not be working. And since they are harder for you, you'll get your heart rate up faster. You always get a better workout practicing your weakest strokes."

Tie one on. Swimming may be an all-body sport, but experts recommend working specific muscles. "One of the best things you can do is tie your legs together so that you just work your arms and shoulders," Stephens says. "You can also strengthen your leg muscles by getting a kickboard and just kicking your way across the pool to improve your kick."

By targeting specific muscle areas, Stephens says that you'll get a more intense workout and burn more calories.

Question your form. To go faster longer, you need proper technique and form. And one of the most common mistakes among recreational swimmers is not using the "S-shaped pull," says Jane Katz, Ed.D., also a "Masters" swimming champion, world-record holder, and the author of seven books on swimming technique, including *The All-American Aquatics Handbook* (1-800-278-3525) and *The New W.E.T. Workout* (1-800-322-8755). "With the S-pull, you're moving your hands underwater in an S-motion during a crawl—your right hand makes a question mark and your left hand makes a reverse question mark."

She acknowledges that while some recreational swimmers do practice the S-pull, most don't. "But if you practice that during your workout, you'll get a better workout because it enhances your swimming technique, it makes swimming more efficient, and you'll be able to go faster and go longer."

Act like Flipper. To improve endurance, some experts suggest that you practice underwater swimming so that your body gets trained to work on less oxygen. To do that, try this drill, recommended by Jane Cappaert,

---

Cross-Training ⤵ Tip

Swimming pools aren't just for swimming anymore.

"Deep-water running is the closest thing you can do to simulate running without the pounding you get from the road," says Doug Stern, a New York City triathlete and swimming author for *Triathlete* magazine who teaches deep-water running at places like the New York Road Runner's Club through his company, Doug Stern Swimming Clinics, also in New York City. "What's more, it gives you a great workout and can actually improve your running performance."

In deep-water running, you wear a life preserver, ski belt, or any type of belt or device that keeps your head above water (there are specific products made for deep-water running, such as the AquaJogger, 1-800-922-9544) and practice "running" in place for up to 45 minutes—with minimal knee bend, toes pointed downward, hands below your elbows, and hips in line with your shoulders.

As you progress, you can practice "hurdle jumping" by reaching forward with your arm to touch your lead foot and "uphill running" by exaggerating the backswing of your elbows and lifting your knees slightly higher. Always practice these techniques in deep water. You also can improve your running technique by being aware of your form. "Form will breed speed," says Stern.

---

director of biomechanics with the U.S. Olympic swimming team in 1992 and 1996. At one side of the pool, take a deep breath and then submerge as you push off the wall with your feet. Hold your arms in front of you, torpedo-like, and move yourself with a dolphin kick, keeping your legs together and outstretched as you move them up and down like a dolphin moves its tail. Once you've crossed the pool in one breath, try to increase your speed.

Tennis

Increase Your Net Worth

Watch the pros on TV and you might think that the hardest workout they get comes from trying to carry home their tournament winnings.

After all, what they consider work—batting around a tennis ball for a couple of hours in Boca Raton—is what we call vacation. Add an adoring Brooke Shields to the scenario and it's a vacation that beats Disney World hands down.

Ace Your Next Workout

Maybe the pros just make it look easy. But even those of us who move more like Boris Karloff than Boris Becker can get a pretty decent workout playing tennis. The average guy burns more than 500 calories in an hour of singles and can get his heart rate to its target zone within a few minutes. That's a better workout than you'd get cycling at a 10-mile-per-hour (mph) pace and about the same as using a rowing machine. And in that hour, even amateur players are hitting the ball at about 50 mph, says Vic Braden, instruction editor of *Tennis* magazine and director of the Vic Braden Tennis College in Coto De Caza, California, compared to the pros, who can smash the 100 mph barrier.

"Despite what a lot of people think, you can get a tremendous workout playing tennis—even in a limited period of time," says Nick Saviano, who has coached many top American players as director of coaching for men's tennis for the U.S. Tennis Association in Key Biscayne, Florida. "In fact, played and trained for correctly, it can be one of the more

demanding sports around." Here's how to put every minute on the court to your advantage.

Be peppy between points. Unlike the pros who have scads of ball boys to fetch their missed shots, the rest of us have to gather our own. So make the most of it. "If you briskly walk to the ball between points, or even jog, you'll keep your heart rate up and get the best workout in the time you spend playing," Braden says. "The biggest complaint about tennis is that the heart rate goes up and down too much, that it doesn't stay up long enough for casual players to get a good workout. The reason is because too many people use the time between points as a break period. You need to keep moving in order to keep your heart rate up."

Aim high. When your shots fall short, so does your workout. "Most people don't hit deep enough because they don't know the physics of air resistance," Braden says. "Most people aim for just above the net tape (the top of the net), which is why their shots tend to fall near the service line (midcourt). But if you aim your shots five feet above the net, the typical player hitting the ball at 50 mph will land the ball 20 inches inside your opponent's baseline—deep enough to play the corners so you give *him* a great workout chasing your shots."

Jog before you play. Many casual "racketeers" rarely last more than a set or two because their bodies get sore too quickly. The reason is that they either fail to stretch before playing or, even worse, stretch immediately after hitting the court.

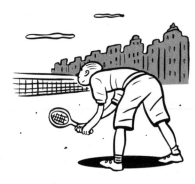

"You should never stretch cold, because you can actually increase your risk of injury. But so many people do it—and that plays a big part in them not getting the most out of their tennis workout," says Braden, who has done extensive biomechanical research with dozens of top-playing professionals, including Jimmy Connors and Chris Evert.

"Your body temperature should be elevated at least three degrees before you begin to stretch your muscles," he says.

To raise your body temperature enough to "warm" muscles for stretching, run around the perimeter of the court two or three times, or just jog in place for about three minutes, says Saviano.

Don't dally when you rally.
"After proper stretching, the best way to enhance your movement, improve your tennis, and get a great workout is to run for every ball," Saviano says. "Too many players let the ball bounce twice in their warm-ups or don't chase balls that they perceive as out of their reach.

"If you go after every ball—whether it's in or out, whether you're warming up or playing a game—you'll get a great aerobic workout and also dramatically improve your footwork and timing," says Saviano.

Be ready to hit. "Another reason why some people don't get a good workout playing tennis is because they make errors too quickly," says Braden. "The longer the ball stays in play, the greater your oxygen demands and the better workout you'll get."

Braden says that most unforced errors and mishit balls result from not having your racket back early enough to receive the ball from your opponent. "Most people wait until the ball has bounced on their side before they bring their racket back to hit the ball. That doesn't leave them enough time to make a good shot. Instead, they should be bringing their rackets back the instant their opponent hits it. Look at the pros and you'll see that they have their rackets back before the ball even crosses over the net," says Braden.

Start your approach earlier. Lazy footwork is another obstacle to maximizing your on-court tennis workout. "You should emphasize moving to the ball as quickly as possible, then take your time on the stroke.

Cross-Training ⚡Tip

As director of coaching for men's tennis for the U.S. Tennis Association—the governing agency of the sport—Nick Saviano has coached some of America's best professional and amateur players on the finer points of tennis. Among their conditioning secrets is playing basketball.

"A lot of players will play basketball to help cross-train for their tennis because they share a lot of the same athletic movements," Saviano says. "It improves hand-eye coordination as well as endurance. And it also involves explosive movements. Plus, basketball is something that you can do by yourself. Just going out and shooting and retrieving the ball can give you a great workout in a short period of time."

Besides basketball, Saviano suggests doing sprints to enhance anaerobic capacity and quickness. "While a lot of players jog—which promotes aerobic conditioning, not quickness—I'd recommend concentrating on doing 220s and 20-yard dashes, especially during the playing season," he says.

This will improve your tennis game and give you a great cardiovascular workout," Saviano says. "One common mistake is that many players get lulled into a false sense of having lots of time when an opponent hits the ball. In order to get a quick first move on his opponent's shot, the player should start his split step as his opponent starts swinging his racket forward to hit the ball," he says. A split step is when a player establishes his balance by taking a little jump off the ground with his feet shoulder-width apart. Landing on his toes with his feet in position, the player can then make a move in any direction. "This enables the player to move even before the ball crosses the net."

Walking

Put Your Best Foot Forward

Those first few steps were exciting enough. Mom cheering and steering you past the furniture as Dad got it all on film with his Kodak Instamatic camera. You were growing up. Going places. And the world was at your feet—literally.

Today, though, walking is no big deal for most guys—even if they do it while chewing gum. In fact, most of us would sooner ask for directions than admit that we walk for fitness. After all, softball offers us camaraderie and beer. Basketball with your buddies allows even the most vertically challenged among us to engage in the fine art of trash talking. But walking? For fitness? That's something for old ladies in shopping malls, right?

Walk This Way

"It's true that walking is not the first choice of exercise for a lot of guys. They may think that because it is a less aggressive sport, that the benefits aren't that great," says Don Lawrence, who conducts walking clinics for NaturalSport Walking Shoes and coaches his wife, Olympic racewalker Debbi Lawrence. "In a sport dominated by women, we are seeing more and more couples walking together. This makes a statement that men today realize the positive results walking has to offer. This activity—walking—adds a calming form of exercise to an already-stress-filled workday. You can take this sport to any level you want," says Lawrence. In fact, in

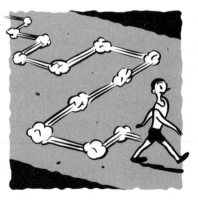

Olympic competition, male racewalkers average under seven minutes per mile for 31 miles—a speed many joggers would be proud to claim.

But what walking lacks in public relations it makes up for in perks. After hundreds of studies, many of the nation's top fitness authorities consider walking to be the perfect way to boost fitness—including Dr. Kenneth Cooper of the Cooper Aerobics Center, who practically single-handedly started America's obsession with running.

That's because walking offers similar calorie-burning and heart and lung–boosting benefits to those gained through running and other aerobic exercises—only with far less damage to your joints. It requires no special equipment or athletic skills, although you probably don't want to do it in your wing tips too often. It can be done anywhere by just about anyone over the age of one.

"And perhaps the best-kept secret of all, it can give you a tremendous workout in a minimum of amount of time," says Casey Meyers, a walking lecturer and author of *Walking: The Complete Guide to the Complete Exercise* and *Aerobic Walking*. Here's how to make the most of your next walking workout.

Make it brisk. "The key for getting the best walking workout, especially when time is short, is very simple," says Meyers, who held walking clinics for the famed Cooper Wellness Program in Dallas for six years and is a frequent talk-show guest on the benefits of walking.

"You need to pick up the pace."

That may sound obvious, but research has shown that moving just a little quicker can bring big results, Meyers says. Walking at an aerobic 12- to 13-minute-per-mile pace—achievable by most reasonably fit men—can *quadruple* aerobic capacity compared to walking at a more leisurely "strolling" pace of 20 minutes per mile, says Meyers. In fact, the quicker pace

can bring you the same aerobic benefits as running the same distance at
about a 9-minute-mile pace, says
Meyers.

"Besides, if you're walking three
miles a day, moving up to a 12- or 13-
minute pace will not only improve
your fitness level but you can also
achieve that improvement in about half
the time of walking the same three
miles at a strolling pace," Meyers says.

Don't overstride. It seems
logical: If you want to cover more
ground fast, take bigger steps. But it
doesn't work that way. "The real trick
to walking faster and getting the best
workout in the shortest time period is
to take more steps per minute than
you usually walk," Lawrence says.
"Too many people think that the key
to walking faster is to take a bigger
stride, but that is less efficient. A
quicker stride can be achieved by
counting your steps in 30 seconds. Develop a rhythm to gradually increase
the steps per minute."

Arm yourself. Your arms are
actually the real key to a better walking
workout, says Martin Rudow of Seattle,
former coach of the men's U.S.
National Racewalking Team. "The correct arm position is crucial in helping
you get a quicker and shorter stride,
which is really the only way to get a
quality workout from walking," he
says. "Arms should be bent at the
elbow at about a 90-degree angle and
should swing close to the body from
the lower breastbone to the back of the
hips. Don't let your arms chicken-wing
out or else you'll throw off your stride."

"Your arms are so important,"
adds Lawrence, "because, when pumped in an
efficient manner, they contribute to overall
body balance and fluidity in motion. Just a
simple technique change like bringing your

Cross-Training Tip

If you're serious about getting the most out of your
walking workout, leave the weights in the gym. And then
set aside time to use them there. Because while walking
and weight lifting at the same time isn't exactly
practical, they do complement each other extremely
well, says Martin Rudow, former coach of the men's U.S.
National Racewalking Team.

"Anything you do that improves your strength and
flexibility will help you become a better walker, but I find
weight lifting to be especially useful," Rudow says. "In
fact, the only way you'll really get a great workout from
walking is with racewalking, and most people don't
realize how important upper-body strength is for
effective racewalking technique. The legs do all the
work, but they follow your arms, so you can go further
and more economically."

That's why Rudow and other elite racewalkers hit
the gym with weights several times a week before
hitting the road. "But I never lift weights for my legs just
to build strength—only for my shoulders, arms, and
chest," he says.

He advises building up the upper body with biceps
and triceps curls for the arms, lateral raises for a
stronger neck and shoulders, and bench and military
presses for the chest muscles. "And while others recommend doing a lot of reps with low weights, I take the
other approach and go for a lot of weight with low reps
to add strength to my upper body," says Rudow.

arms up to a 90-degree angle can add speed to
your walking."

Take the straight and narrow. Most
recreational walkers do what's called

railroading—walking with their legs shoulder-width apart or more, as though they were on the rails of a train track. "The proper form for race-walking or even fast walking is to walk with your feet in a straight line, or close to it," says Lawrence. "That means that if you drew a line on the ground, your left and right foot would be in that line. This is achieved by centering your walking form around your power source—the midsection and hips. This also propels your body forward so that you are able to walk at a faster rate."

Forget the weights. Wearing ankle weights or carrying hand weights won't give you a better workout. In fact, they cause imbalances in your body that can slow you down and increase your risk of joint injuries—a rarity in fitness walking.

"What's more, studies show that in order to make hand weights useful, you'd have to wildly swing your arms in a goofy manner, which changes the rhythm of your walk. Proper arm swinging counterbalances your leg swing," Meyers says.

Be daring on the downhill. You'll get a better workout if you include hills on your walking route. "There's no question that walking up a hill, you don't have to walk as fast to get the heart rate up and get a better workout," Meyers says. "Unfortunately, unless you're on a treadmill, you usually have to turn around and walk down the hill. And most people do it at their normal pace or even slower than usual, which makes it hard to keep your heart rate up. So if you're going down a hill, you need to really pick up the pace and go as fast as possible in order to maintain an elevated heart rate."

Get a leg up. Many guys think that killer quads are the cornerstone of a powerful stride, but, truth be told, it's all of your leg

On Your Marx . . .

If the weather outside is fit for neither man nor beast, you can step onto a treadmill and actually build muscle while you walk. There's only one caveat: You have to walk like Groucho Marx.

Groucho's exaggerated gait is actually a lunge, "one of the best exercises that you can do to strengthen the lower body," says Scott Roberts, Ph.D., author of *Fitness Walking*. Doing lunges on a treadmill gives your thigh and calf muscles a potent strength workout.

Here's how to do it: Adjust the treadmill to a three- to four-degree incline and set the speed for 1 to 1.5 miles per hour. (For safety, never exceed 1.5 miles per hour.) Now extend your arms in front of you so that your forearms rest on the safety bar. With your back straight, take a giant step forward with your right foot. (*Note:* You may need to take shorter strides if you find yourself slipping off the treadmill's belt.) Bend your right knee until your thigh is almost parallel with the floor. (*Caution:* Make sure that your kneecap never extends beyond your front foot, a mistake that can strain ligaments.) As your right foot passes underneath you, step with your left leg and lunge so that your left thigh becomes parallel with the floor. Continue lunge-walking for 60 seconds, then rest for a minute by walking normally on the treadmill. Repeat the exercise 8 to 10 more times.

muscles that help you walk longer, stronger, and faster. "Walking is a total leg workout. As the leg swings forward, the quads contract at heel strike. If the leg is straight, the hamstrings engage and the pull-through is generated by the muscles in the back of the leg," Lawrence says. "The push-off calls upon the calf, hamstring, and buttocks muscles to power your stride forward."

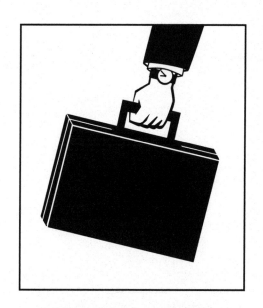

Part Three

Making Time

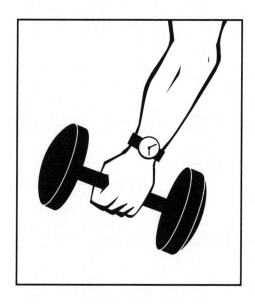

The Best Time for Exercise

Find What Works for You

Everybody, even *your* body, follows a daily rhythm, a circadian rhythm. This physiological clock governs most of the bodily functions we take for granted—what time you sleep and wake up, when you're feeling most alert, when you're most susceptible or resistant to pain or illness, even when you're at the peak of physical ability. Eons of evolution, coupled with our own unique chemistry and daily routine, conspire to set our body clocks.

"The more you understand how your clock works, the more you can work with it for better mental and physical health, and the less you'll do something to disrupt it," says Phyllis Zee, M.D., Ph.D., director of the sleep disorders program at Northwestern University Medical School in Chicago and an expert on biological rhythms.

And believe us, you don't want to go messing with the hands of your body clock. "The things we do or don't do during the day can alter our circadian rhythms, and that can have ramifications on all your body functions— from heart rhythms to bowel function to athletic performance," Dr. Zee says.

For better or worse, here are a few items that may change your body clock.

• Drugs. Caffeine, anti-histamines, alcohol, sleeping pills, and numerous other drugs that liven or deaden our bodies can also affect circadian rhythm. "I wouldn't advise taking these an hour before bed, for example," Dr. Zee says. "They can all disrupt sleep patterns, which, in turn, will cause problems with your circadian rhythms." Yes, that goes for sleeping pills, too. "Unless your doctor has prescribed them, I would avoid sleeping aids," Dr. Zee says.

• Stress. This is one of the most common causes of body-clock disruption, especially where your sleep cycle is concerned. "And it's not just the stress but also stress-relieving medications that we might take," Dr. Zee says. "It's a vicious cycle." All the more reason to adopt a regular workout routine—nothing bashes stress like exercise.

• Sex. Luckily, sex isn't detrimental to your body rhythms. In fact, as most men know and most women lament, a little sex can make you drowsy after the fact. Having sex before bedtime is one of the surest ways we know for getting to sleep quickly and soundly.

• Travel. Few factors are more vexing to your body's cycle than travel. "It's a frequent cause of body-rhythm disruption, especially when traveling through a couple different time zones," Dr. Zee says. Suddenly, it's light when it should be dark, and you're eating when you should be sleeping. The best way to minimize jet lag is to try to get up and go to bed as close to your home time as possible when you're away, says Adele Pace, M.D., a fitness consultant in Ashland, Kentucky, and author of *The Busy Executive's Guide to Total Fitness.*

Working 'round the Clock

Now that you understand a little about your biological rhythms, it's time to apply that knowledge to the task of exercise.

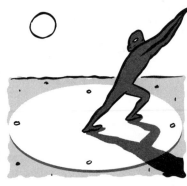

"There are certain times of the day where you're going to be better equipped to perform certain tasks," says Dr. Zee. For example, there are periods throughout the day when our eyesight is sharper, our ability to handle complex mental problems is increased, or our bodies are most receptive to different types of exercise.

But the best time for you to

work out is not entirely at the whim of your body clock, says Dr. Pace. "Attitude plays a big role. You may have spent your whole life thinking that you're an evening person, and nothing on earth could get you out of bed for a 6:00 A.M. run. But until you try it, you'll never know. It may be the perfect thing to wake you up, clear the mental cobwebs, and get you ready for the day," she says.

So experiment a little. Rest assured, whatever type of exercise you want to do, there's a perfect time of day for it. Here's how to find that time and make the most of it.

Exercise early. As with any workout routine, you'll want to identify your goals before picking a time to work out. Think about what you want to accomplish.

"If you're looking to have a regular, consistent routine, then you're better off adopting a morning program," says John Amberge, a certified strength and conditioning specialist and director of corporate programs for the Sports Training Institute in New York City. As Amberge explains, you can get your exercise in first thing, before you're distracted or tired later in the day and get thrown off your schedule.

Biologically, this isn't when your body is at its most powerful, but it's still pretty well equipped to deal with exercise. Dr. Zee says that in the morning, a man's body is naturally firing off bursts of testosterone, which help maintain muscle mass. It's also pumping cortisol, a hormone that helps us deal with mental and physical stress. Plus, our temperature is rising from an evening of sleep, priming the pump for physical activity.

Perform in the afternoon. If you're preparing for an endurance event or are doing serious weight training where you're trying to push the envelope or break out of a weight-training plateau, then you'll probably want to find time to exercise in the afternoon.

"Several studies show that we tend to be stronger and perform better in the afternoon," Dr. Zee says. "Our grip strength is stronger, and muscle tone improves."

Lighten up in the evening. If you're in reasonably good shape or are just beginning an exercise program, your needs may be lighter, in which case, you can do your workout in the evening.

"Evening is probably the time when you'll best respond to light exercise," says Amberge. It'll minimize the impact of a heavy dinner, and light exercise can actually help you rest easier. "It might be just enough to tire you out so that you'll sleep like a baby," says Amberge.

Making the Right Time

Beyond the biological imperatives, there are ways that you can actively nail down the best time for you to exercise.

"To some degree, it's not a question of finding time but making time," says Virginia Bass, time-management consultant for Day-Timers in Exton, Pennsylvania. "That's when you have to take a hard look at the daily routine that you—not Mother Nature—have established for yourself. Then, you have to find a way to insert exercise into that routine." Here's how to do it.

Check your appointment book. The first, most obvious step is to review your schedule over the course of the average week.

"Take note of the times you consistently have open. Typically, those are going to be in the morning, at lunch, or after work, but a lot of men have other gaps in their daily schedule," Bass says. For example, you may never have anything going from 11:00 A.M. to 12:00 noon or from 2:45 P.M. to 3:30 P.M. That's time that you might be able to devote to getting some exercise.

Work on flextime. Many businesses offer flextime hours. As long as you work your 40 hours a week and are working during core business hours (typically 10:00 A.M. to 4:00 P.M.), when you arrive and leave can be a gray area worth exploiting.

"If you've been working 9:00 A.M. to 5:00 P.M. all your life and you haven't found time for

Clock Wise

Are you a night owl, a lark, or something in between? Take our quiz and find out.

After reading each of the following questions, circle the number that follows the response that best describes you. Add up the numbers to get your score and compare it to the scale at the end of the quiz.

1. If you were free to plan your day, when would you get up and when would you go to bed?

Get up (A.M.)
5 to 6:30 **5**   6:31 to 7:45 **4**   7:46 to 9:45 **3**   9:46 to 11:00 **2**   11:01 to noon **1**

Go to bed (P.M.)
8 to 9 **5**   9:01 to 10:15 **4**   10:16 to 12:30 **3**   12:31 to 1:45 **2**   1:46 to 3 **1**

2. If you have to get up at a specific time, how dependent are you on the alarm clock to wake you?

Not at all dependent **4**   Slightly dependent **3**   Fairly dependent **2**   Very dependent **1**

3. How easy is getting up in the morning?

Not at all easy **1**   Not very easy **2**   Fairly easy **3**   Very easy **4**

4. During the first half-hour after waking up . . .

How alert are you?
Not at all **1**   Slightly **2**   Fairly **3**   Very **4**

How tired are you?
Very tired **1**   Fairly tired **2**   Fairly refreshed **3**   Very refreshed **4**

How's your appetite?
Very poor **1**   Fairly poor **2**   Fairly good **3**   Very good **4**

5. If you have no commitments the next day, when do you go to bed compared with your usual bedtime?

Seldom or never later **4**   1 to 2 hours later **2**
Less than 1 hour later **3**   More than 2 hours later **1**

6. Some friends want you to exercise hard with them. How would you perform . . .

From 7 to 8 A.M.?
Quite well **4**   Reasonably well **3**   Poorly **2**   Very poorly **1**

exercise, maybe what you need to do is alter your schedule. See if you can work from 7:30 A.M. to 3:30 P.M. or from 10:00 A.M. to 6:00 P.M. All of a sudden, you have extra time in the morning or evening that you can devote entirely to a workout," Bass says. "It never hurts to check with your manager or personnel office to see if this is possible."

Exercise morning, noon, and night.
For the moment, forget what your body clock tells you and what your schedule demands of you. Never mind whether you think you're a morning person or a night person. If you're just getting started on an exercise program, the first thing that you should do is exercise at different times of the day.

From 10 to 11 P.M.?

Quite well **1**   Reasonably well **2**   Poorly **3**   Very poorly **4**

7. When in the evening are you tired and ready for bed?

8 to 9 P.M. **5**   9:01 to 10:15 P.M. **4**   10:16 P.M. to 12:45 A.M. **3**

12:46 to 2 A.M. **2**   2:01 to 3 A.M. **1**

8. When would you be at your peak for:

A grueling two-hour quiz?

8 to 10 A.M. **6**   11 A.M. to 1 P.M. **4**   3 to 5 P.M. **2**   7 to 9 P.M. **0**

Two hours of exhausting physical work?

8 to 10 A.M. **4**   11 A.M. to 1 P.M. **3**   3 to 5 P.M. **2**   7 to 9 P.M. **1**

9. You've gone to bed several hours later than usual, but you can wake up when you wish to. What is most likely to happen?

You'll wake up at the usual time and stay awake   **4**
You'll wake up at the usual time and doze lightly   **3**
You'll wake up at the usual time but fall back asleep   **2**
You'll wake up later than usual   **1**

10. One morning you must be on watch from 4 to 6 A.M. You have no commitments the rest of the day. Which of the following would you do?

Would not go to bed until watch was over   **1**
Would take a nap before watch and sleep after   **2**
Would take a good sleep before watch and nap after   **3**
Would take all sleep before watch   **4**

Now add up your score.

Score (total points) _____

Score

14–23	**Night owl**	**32–44**	**Intermediate type**	**53–65**	**Lark (morning type)**
24–31	**Almost an owl**	**45–52**	**Almost a lark**		

"Everyone's different. And if you've never exercised regularly before, you really have no idea what time will feel right for you to exercise," says Amberge.

For the first couple weeks, try getting up earlier and exercising before you go to work. Then, try exercising at lunch. Then, try working out after work. If at any point you find a time that really works for you—where you really feel on top of it, or you reach the point where you even enjoy exercise—then stick with it.

If none of these three time periods works, try working out at odd, alternating times—10:30 A.M., 2:00 P.M., 8:00 P.M. "Sooner or later, you'll hit on the right combination," Amberge says.

Working Out in the Morning

How to Be a Rising Son

Ah, the crack of dawn. If you're one of those rare breed of men, it's a time when you bounce out of bed prepared for exercise, feeling clear-eyed, sharp-minded, and ready to give the world a right swift kick in the pants. In which case, you won't need any help from this chapter.

But if you're like most guys, you view the morning through a sleep-encrusted haze that only a shower, a belt of coffee, and a few hours of being upright will cure. On top of that, morning can be a study in hurried chaos. Ties stubbornly refuse to knot themselves; socks that were there a moment ago have suddenly gone AWOL. For that matter, so have your wallet and keys. There's a logjam in the bathroom or the kitchen, and that's only a prelude to what you'll find on the roads as you start your long trip to work. Is this a time to be working out? No, you think, surely not.

That's not how exercise experts view the morning. In fact, they see the morning hours as the best time for a busy man's workout.

Action in the A.M.

"There's real value in working out in the morning. It's a much quieter time of the day—you'll be less likely to be distracted or interrupted in your workout. It'll wake you up; you'll feel more alert driving to work. And that will carry into work, too," says fitness consultant Dr. Adele Pace.

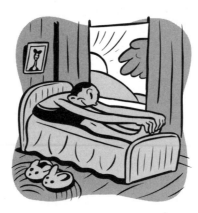

Moreover, once you've done your workout, you don't have to worry about exercising again for the rest of the day (unless you really want to). "That's a tremendous advantage right there," says John Amberge of the Sports Training Institute. "I work with a lot of busy executives, and nothing gives them more enthusiasm about their jobs and themselves than getting right up and exercising. Then, they're done—they don't have to worry about some emergency coming up that's going to prevent them from exercising later."

More Time, Less Risk

Now, perhaps you've heard the news reports that there's a greater risk of heart attack in the morning, a risk you might increase by exercising.

"There's some truth to morning heart attack risk," Dr. Pace says. "But it's not enough to justify not exercising." As Dr. Pace explains, in the morning, certain elements in our blood have a greater tendency to clump together. "In some cases, this can cause a blood clot, which leads to a heart attack." But the men who are at the greatest risk for that kind of health risk are the ones who don't exercise regularly. If your doctor has okayed you to exercise, then you should have no problem working out in the morning.

"The trick is to give yourself plenty of time in the morning so that you can start slow and allow your body—which has been lying inert for six to seven hours—to gradually shift into an exercise mode," Amberge says. But first, you have to learn how to plan a morning exercise routine, then make sure that you stick to it. Here's your wake-up call.

Turn back the clock.
Before you can have a workout, you have to make time for that

workout. The best way to do it is to lay hands on that bedside clock and set it to go off 15 minutes earlier. Give yourself a week or two to get used to your new time, then set it back another 15 minutes. "Now you've added a half-hour to your day, and you can devote it purely to exercise," says Dr. Pace.

Just be sure to give yourself time to adjust to your new schedule. "Don't set the clock back a half-hour or more the first week. That's too harsh on your system. Give yourself time to adjust," says Dr. Pace.

Turn in earlier. If you're committed to a morning routine, don't expect to be able to go to bed at midnight like you used to. "If you're getting up earlier, you're going to have to go to bed earlier. Some people have a problem with that," Dr. Pace says. "But really, you're better off going to bed earlier than watching bad TV and eating late-night snacks."

Do it yesterday. Think about your morning routine: You clamber out of bed, soak in the shower, root through your closet for a tie to match your shirt, then stumble downstairs to make a pot of coffee. If you're thrifty, maybe you make a lunch and head out the door. What a waste of time.

"If you look at your morning schedule with an eye toward saving time, you'll probably see dozens of little things that you could do the night before to give yourself more time for exercise in the morning," says Virginia Bass of Day-Timers. "Buying a coffeemaker with a timer that you can set at night; making a lunch; setting your keys, wallet, and briefcase by the door so that you don't have to look for them." All of these will save you minutes in the morning—and it only takes a few minutes to add another set of reps or another mile to your workout.

Top of the Morning

The envelope, please. And the winner in the category of "Best Morning Exercise" is . . . running.

"If you already run, you know that it can be a great way to start the morning off," says fitness consultant Dr. Adele Pace.

One caution: If you've never run before, get your doctor's approval first. And even then, start out slowly. For the first week, just walk. Then mix walking with brief spurts of running, says Dr. Pace. After a month, you'll be able to run around the neighborhood to your heart's content.

That said, the morning is prime time for running. Let us count the ways.

It's cool. Even on the hottest summer days, morning is the coolest time. You'll still get a good workout, but it will be easier on your heart, says Dr. Pace.

There's less. Less traffic, that is. Fewer people, too. "You'll be less likely to be distracted or interrupted. You can sort out your plans for the day," says John Amberge of the Sports Training Institute.

The air is fresh. "Pollution is at its lowest levels before rush hour in the morning," notes Dr. Pace. Less pollution means less poisons that you'll absorb while running. The less you absorb, the less your likelihood of developing cancer.

Adopt a dress code. Clothing is another night-before task—both the outfit you wear to work and the one you'll wear to work out in.

"Go to bed in shorts and a T-shirt or, if it's cold, sweatpants and a T-shirt. Then, when the alarm goes off, you get up, jump into your sneakers, and you're ready to go," Bass says.

As far as your work wardrobe goes, match your tie to your shirt before you go to bed (you can even tie it, loosen it enough to get it over your head, and leave it on a hanger until morning). Or if you work out at a club, have your work clothes packed and in the car, ready to go in the morning.

Don't shower. If you plan to work out at a health club before work, don't jump in the shower at home before you head out.

"You're better off waiting until you get to the club," says Amberge. Too many would-be exercisers decide to blow the club off in the crush of traffic. Unless you're intent on career suicide, your smelly unbathed self will be a powerful incentive to make sure that you stop at the club to bathe. And heck, as long as you're stopping at the club for a shower, you might as well get your money's worth and hit a few of the machines, right?

Avoid weekend weakness. "One of the best things you can do to stay on an exercise schedule is to get up and go to bed at the same time every day, even on the weekends," Dr. Pace says. "Sleeping in on weekends—and I mean sleeping in by more than an hour—is just going to throw the whole routine off." So once you have your timing down, stick with it. Your reward will be a body and mind that will function smoothly—almost like clockwork.

Making the Most of Morning

Now that you've cordoned off a chunk of the morning for a workout, it's time to make sure that your workout is the most effective one possible.

"Whether you're doing an aerobic exercise or weight training in the basement, there are several performance and safety issues to remember," says Barry Franklin, Ph.D., director of cardiac rehabilitation and exercise laboratories at William Beaumont Hospital Rehabilitation and Health Center in Birmingham, Michigan. By following these precepts, you'll make sure that

your body is operating at peak efficiency, which will not only make the most of your workout but also help you avoid injury. Start your morning this way.

Drink early and often. Although it's a good idea to drink plenty of fluids before you exercise, it's doubly important in the morning. "Think about it—it's been several hours since you drank anything—you could be dehydrated and not even know it," says Amberge. So before you hit the weight bench, hit the sink and quaff a couple glasses of water.

Ease into it. Another regular aspect of exercise that takes on extra importance in the morning is your warm-up sequence. "The importance of a warm-up cannot be overemphasized," Dr. Franklin says. "Jumping out of bed and starting a workout may be too hard on the body and especially hard on the heart." Instead, spend a good 10 minutes doing light exercise—some calisthenics, running in place, mild stretching, a brisk walk around the neighborhood—anything to prepare for heavier exercise.

Be cool. Once you've completed your workout of choice, don't make the mistake of coming to an abrupt stop. "That's also hard on the heart. That's why it's just as important to do some cooldown exercises after a workout," says Dr. Franklin. A light walk, some stretching, a few calisthenics—all are excellent cooldown choices.

Eat your breakfast. Once you've completed your workout, make sure that you eat a good breakfast. "When people are trying to make time for exercise in the morning, one area they often cut time out of is their breakfast time. It's a mistake. You need your breakfast," Dr. Pace says. So eat it. But shy away from the heavy, fattening foods—eggs, bacon, doughnuts, to name a few. Instead, stick with bagels and jelly, low-fat yogurt, whole-grain breads, and cereals.

"After a workout, your muscles are going to be crying for fuel. These foods all have carbohydrates—the fuel that both your body and your brain need," Amberge says.

Commuter Calisthenics

Developing a Rush-Hour Routine

Like waiting in a doctor's office or number punching your way through a voice-mail maze, commuting is one of life's necessary wastes of time. You don't get where you need to be without an unenviable and inconvenient delay.

In the world of commuting, that delay is pretty significant. According to government estimates, the average worker spends nearly 40 minutes a day commuting if he travels by car. If he takes a bus, he's looking at more than an hour round-trip; and if he rides the rails, his commute averages more than two hours a day.

To those of us trying to make time for exercise, these statistics certainly seem daunting. Imagine if you could do a two-hour workout every morning instead of sitting on a train. Until someone invents a Star Trek–style transporter, you figure, your chances of turning commuting time into exercise time are slim.

But not impossible.

Training in Transit

Whether it's by car, bus, or train, there are numerous ways to turn some of those lost morning and evening commuting hours into workout time.

"No matter what mode of travel you use, there's probably some way to convert a bit of your commuting time into exercise time," assures John Amberge of the Sports Training Institute.

"It won't be anything like a good workout in the gym, of course. But if you can steal five minutes a day for exercise, that's almost an extra half-hour of exercise a week." Such time makes a great supplement to your regular routine, he adds.

As a first step toward commuter calisthenics, start paying attention to the gaps in your commuting time, says Sandra Lotz Fisher, exercise physiologist and president of New York City's Fitness by Fisher, a fitness and stress-management consulting firm. "When you're waiting for your ride, anytime you're a passenger in a vehicle, when you're at a stoplight, while you're in a traffic jam—these are all times that you can devote to a variety of exercises without endangering yourself or your fellow commuters." No matter how you get to work, we have an exercise plan for you.

The Freeway to Fitness

For those of us who commute by car, it seems like there's no way to exercise en route—not without ending up on the Eye-in-the-Sky traffic report as the accident that's blocking the left lane.

"Not so," says Fisher, who developed "Freeway Flex: Stretch and Tone Exercises to Do While You Drive," an audio exercise tape designed especially for motorists, available from Fitness by Fisher by calling (212) 744-5900. But, she cautions, "you absolutely shouldn't do it at any point where it's going to take your attention off the road."

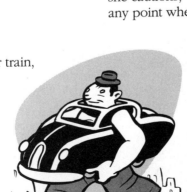

That said, if you drive in light to moderate conditions, there's plenty of time during your morning or evening drive that you can convert to exercise time.

"Gridlock can be your friend," says Charles Kuntzleman, Ed.D., professor of kinesiology at the University of Michigan in Ann Arbor and director of Blue Cross and Blue Shield of Michigan Fitness for Youth Program, also at the University of Michigan. Basically, anytime that traffic is at a standstill, that's time you can spend doing a few simple exercises—instead of getting frustrated about a backup."

Our experts have provided a few in-car exercises to be performed while waiting in traffic—not while driving—that will help you use traffic time constructively and avoid rear-ending someone out of sheer frustration.

Just shrug. Shoulder shrugs are a good tension reliever and exercise for shoulder and arm muscles. Grip the wheel at the nine and three o'clock positions, and push back against your seat until your arms are straight. Now raise your shoulders up toward your ears. Do 10, or as many as you can until traffic starts moving, Dr. Kuntzleman says.

Keep your hands on the wheel.
Simply squeeze the steering wheel as hard as you can. Hold for a count of five, then relax. "Really focus on the release part," Dr. Kuntzleman says. "That stimulates a relaxation response in the body, which will help you be more loose and limber when you get to work or head to the gym." Although Dr. Kuntzleman suggests this as a way to relieve traffic-induced stress, it's also a good grip strengthener.

Vacuum inside your car. You can't do crunches in a car, but you can still work your abs by doing vacuums, Dr. Kuntzleman says. Sit up straight in your seat. Now, suck in your stomach as though you were on a beach and the Swedish Bikini Team was strolling by. Hold that pose for a count of 10, then relax. Try to do 5 reps, building up to 10.

Take advantage of flex time.
Between brake pumping and gas stomping, at least one leg gets a pretty good workout in the car. Work the other one, too, by doing this thigh-toning, isometric exercise. Tighten your free leg as hard as you can for three seconds, feeling the tightness in your quadriceps and hamstring, and then release. To keep your feet limber, flex your ankle and curl your toes occasionally. "You won't have nearly the cramps and sore leg problems a lot of drivers complain about," Fisher says.

Power on the Platform

Transportation schedules being what they are—that is to say, inaccurate—odds are that you find yourself waiting for your ride a few times a week. That time can be exercise time, whether you're waiting for a train, a bus, or your carpool pals. Don't just sit and page through the paper. Get up and get moving. Here are a few suggestions for waiting games you can play.

Pace like a lion. It drives your wife nuts at home, but she's not here, is she? So burn up some nervous energy while you're waiting for your ride.

"If it's a bus stop, walk up to the corner and back to the stop. Try to do 10 laps before the bus arrives. If it's a train station, try to do as many brisk, walking laps around the station as you can before your train pulls in," suggests Amberge. Anytime you're standing still is time that you can spend doing some exercise.

Do a bus-stop stretch. Dr. Kuntzleman says that most men don't stretch as much as they should. Use your waiting time to get in some light limbering exercises. See that chain-link fence near your bus stop? Stand facing away from it, stretch your arms out behind you, hook your hands into the fence (at about chest level), and lean forward, stretching both your arms and shoulders.

Heel thyself. Another exercise you can do on any city street is a heel raise. Stand on the edge of the curb with your heels hanging off the edge. Now slowly raise yourself up on your toes, then lower yourself (you may want to rest one hand on a handy parking meter or signpost for balance).

Run to catch the train. If you commute by train or subway, it's instinctive to try to position yourself so that, when the train stops, the doors open right in front of you.

"When you think about it, that's really pretty lazy of you," says Fisher. Instead, as the train comes to a complete stop, walk briskly toward the front or the back of the train, whichever is farthest away. You'll get a quick burst of exercise from the activity, and you may find that you'll get on the train faster than if you try to squeeze in with the rest of the throng at the doors in the middle of the train.

Working Out on the Way

Once you're on your way to work or home, you still have plenty of time for exercise, especially if you take public transportation.

"If you're not doing the driving and you're not packed in like sardines, then you have time and space to do some exercise," Fisher says. Here are some ideas to get you started.

Get out and walk. Both Dr. Kuntzleman and Fisher suggest cutting your commute short by at least one stop if it's within several blocks of work. "Before you get to the office, just get out one stop early and walk or run the rest of the way," Dr. Kuntzleman says. "The way traffic is in most cities, you'll probably get there faster on foot." Just remember to wear walking or running shoes—those executive wing tips weren't meant for exercise.

Stand and deliver. If we're on a train or bus, most of us usually search for a seat that we can nab. Don't bother, says Dr. Kuntzleman.

"Unless you have some back problems or a condition that prevents you from standing for long periods of time, you'll get more exercise from simply standing," he says. The swaying of a bus or train causes muscles to fire in your legs, back, torso—even your arms—to help you keep balance. "It's not much, but it's better than sitting and doing nothing," Dr. Kuntzleman says.

Hang out. "If your bus or isn't too crowded, grab a rail or handle on either side of the aisle and lean forward, then back-

Drive, He Said

So driving isn't how you get to work. It *is* your work. Here are three exercises suggested by Marge Rodgers, a physical therapist and rehabilitation services coordinator for Genesis Rehabilitation Services in Baltimore, that will help keep you on the road to good health.

Loosen up. Because tight hamstrings can lead to both knee and back pain, it pays to keep them loose—even if you're sitting behind the wheel of a tractor trailer all day. Before you hit the road, stand by the side of your truck facing the door and lift your foot up and rest your heel on the step with your knee straight but not flexed. This should create a gentle bend in your hamstring—and begin to reduce your chances for back problems.

Roll with it. Crunches are fine, of course, but they're tough to do in a car or truck. So at the next traffic light, give this exercise a try. Slump down in the chair and then lift your chest and push your abs out. "Roll forward, roll back, find your middle, and do an isometric contraction and hold it. Relax. Roll forward, roll back, until you get a good feel for where that middle is, and then do another isometric contraction," Rodgers says. "These muscles need to be strong to help support your spine."

Bend over backward. "Every time you get out of the cab, step to the side of the truck, put your hands on your hips and bend backward, keeping your knees straight," says Rodgers. "This alleviates the stress that's been building in your back while you were sitting hunched forward, creates some space between the disks of your spine, and allows hydration."

ward, stretching your chest and shoulder muscles. It's probably safest to do that anytime the vehicle comes to a stop," Dr. Kuntzleman says.

The Real Power Lunch

Molding Muscles at Midday

Okay, so maybe working out at lunchtime isn't your first choice, but it just may be the best time for you to squeeze in a little exercise.

"Think about it. How long does it take you to eat your lunch—not wolf it down, but casually eat it? Probably 15 minutes, tops," figures fitness consultant Dr. Adele Pace, author of *The Busy Executive's Guide to Total Fitness.*

If you get an hour for lunch, that leaves you 45 minutes of exercise time. That's time enough for a good workout, even if you never leave the confines of your office building.

Although it's right in the middle of the day, lunchtime actually tends to be a popular time for busy guys to exercise, says John Amberge of the Sports Training Institute. "It's a great way to recharge your batteries after a hard morning, and that pick-me-up can carry through the rest of the day."

Making It Work

Cramming a lunchtime workout into your schedule is eminently doable, says Amberge.

"If your exercise facilities are within 10 minutes of your office, you have plenty of time to work out and eat lunch," he says. "We get a lot of executives in here at around 11:30 A.M. They work out for a half-hour to 45 minutes, then they grab lunch on the way back to the office."

Maybe that's not an option for you; maybe your office is miles from a club; or maybe your job demands that you be close by, just in case. Well, you can always work out in the office. If you do, that's almost better, in a way. Since you don't have to go anywhere, you'll have even more time for more exercise.

"Of course, if you exercise around the office, you'll probably want to modify your workout a little bit. You'll want to do enough so that you feel like you're getting some benefit from the activity, but not so much that you end up all sweaty going into your afternoon meetings," says Amberge.

Whatever type of exercise you have time for, heed the following advice. These tips should help you make the most of your midday muscle building.

Drink before noon. Even before the lunch whistle blows, you can start preparing for exercise by making sure that you have plenty of fluids in your system.

"If you're not well-hydrated, it may adversely affect your performance," says Dr. Barry Franklin of William Beaumont Hospital Rehabilitation and Health Center. "You won't be able to make the most of your workout time. I definitely recommend getting some fluids into you." And he means water, not coffee.

The caffeine in coffee will actually cause your body to get rid of more fluids, not to mention the fact that caffeine can increase stress on your heart, Dr. Franklin says. "A couple cups in the morning is fine. But after that, switch to water."

Munch at mid-morning. Roughly an hour before you exercise, start fueling for your workout. "If you're doing any kind of serious weight training or heavy exercise, do not eat lunch before you do it. You'll be too loaded down with food—you'll feel awful," Amberge says. But you have to have some fuel in you, so he

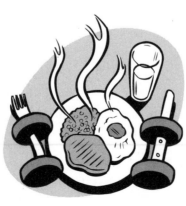

recommends eating something easy to digest but high in carbohydrates, such as a bagel or a piece of fruit.

Eat afterward. After your workout, your body will practically be starving for more fuel. And chances are that you'll be feeling hungrier, so go ahead and eat your lunch afterward. Just be sure that your heart rate is out of its aerobic zone, says Joanne Curran-Celentano, R.D., Ph.D., associate professor of nutrition and food science at the University of New Hampshire in Durham. She suggests that you cool down enough so that your heart rate is close to normal before you eat a full meal. (For a better idea of what to eat, see Packing a Lunch That Packs a Punch on page 120.)

Take a stroll. If you did make it to the gym, odds are that you didn't have time to do much of a cooldown. So before you get back to the office to eat or resume work, walk an easy lap or two around the parking lot.

"It'll be a lot easier on your body—especially your heart and the muscles you just worked out—if you go for a walk or do some light stretching in your office than if you go back upstairs and sit still for the next four to five hours," says Dr. Pace.

Consolidate your efforts. Even if the gym is across the street, you may find yourself crunched for time, between changing, exercising, changing back, showering, *and* eating lunch. So cut some corners. When you work out, stick to a five-minute warm-up and do lifts that only work compound muscle groups—squats, for example, work several muscles at once, says Amberge. For more information on the best workout in the shortest amount of time, see the Ultimate Workout chapters in this book, starting on page 44.

Strictly Business

For years, you've wined and dined your clients. How about slimming and toning them instead?

John Amberge of the Sports Training Institute says you can mix business and exercise. Here's how.

Schedule meetings at the gym. If you have an in-house exercise facility or company membership at a local club, skip the conference room and head straight to the gym.

"If it's just two or three of you and you all work out on a semi-regular basis, just meet there," Amberge says. "You can have a discussion on the stair-climbing machines as easily as you can sitting around a conference table. Then you can all go out for lunch afterward."

Play your client's game. So your weeks of cold calls have finally snagged you a meeting with the executive vice-president of purchasing for ThingamaBob, Inc. Instead of stupefying him with a big lunch, impress him with your athletic ability. "It's no different than meeting someone for golf and conducting business that way," Amberge says. "Only instead of golf, you meet for racquetball or tennis, whatever his favorite game is."

Set an example. So your client doesn't have a favorite activity. Invite him to participate in yours.

Even if he's not into exercise, chances are that your approach will stand out from the pile of business-lunch invitations that he gets all the time.

Bring your own. If you're really serious about working out where you work, bring in a pair of dumbbells and keep them in your office—10- to 15-pounders ought to do nicely. "Then there's any number of arm, shoulder, and chest exercises that you can do right in your own office chair," Amberge says. These range from basic curls to overhead presses. Whatever exercise you choose, you're bound to give new meaning to the term *power lunch*.

The Office Circuit

Unfortunately, all too many guys find themselves with some time to exercise at lunch but not enough to get to a gym and do a serious workout. That's okay. It doesn't mean that you can't get in some exercise at lunch anyway.

"There are a number of exercises that you can do at lunch right around your office, if you want to be creative about it," Amberge says. It doesn't take a lot of extra planning, just a willingness to do it. Most important, you won't break such a sweat that you'll be offending everyone when you walk into an afternoon meeting. Amberge, who helps corporations set up their own in-house exercise programs, suggests the following office circuit. See if you can complete it.

Note: On days when you plan to do an office workout—or any workout where you're on your feet—it pays to pack along a pair of walking shoes or cross-trainers. Your feet will thank you.

Warm-Up

This may be a fairly low-intensity exercise program, but it still pays to warm up your muscles before you use them. Here's how.

Visit your vehicle. You remembered to park your car at the furthest reaches of the lot and walk in, didn't you? Now, walk out to it, briskly, with a little bit of swing in your arms. From your desk chair to the driver's seat and back is one lap. Do at least two laps.

Walk the halls. Now do one circuit around the perimeter of the floor your office is located on.

Working Around the Working Lunch

Sooner or later it's going to happen: Your boss will storm into your office and announce that you and the rest of the department will be having a "working lunch" in the dungeon conference room today. Or maybe you're locked in to a big business lunch at that overpriced Italian place down the street, and there's no getting out of it. Either way, your lunchtime plans for a workout are shot, and there's no way you can make it up tonight or tomorrow morning.

Relax. If your only time to exercise has suddenly been compromised by the necessities of professional life, a modicum of damage control will see you through. Here's some advice to help you over the working-lunch hump.

Double up. Often, you know about these meetings in advance, says fitness consultant Dr. Adele Pace. Review your schedule at the beginning of the week. If you have a business lunch coming up—or see a meeting that could spill over into your workout time at lunch—you can take precautionary measures.

"Spend a few extra minutes the day before and the day after on your workout. Or make the day before a high-tempo day when you're going to push yourself. Set the stair-climbing machine at a higher level than you normally do for

"You can even mix it up with some interval training; sprint for a couple of seconds, then slow back down to a brisk walk," suggests Amberge. Time those sprints so that you'll be dashing past the boss's office—you'll look like you're rushing to an important meeting, at lunch no less!—and you might even boost your career health, too.

Workout

Now that you're warmed up, you're ready to get down to business. Try these exercises.

a few intervals. Add on an extra set to some of your lifts," she says. "This way, missing a workout the next day gives you the rest you need to recover. You've gained, not lost."

Cut your losses. Just because you can't exercise doesn't mean that you can't treat your body well at the restaurant. Make smart choices. Order a big salad, and avoid the heavy slabs of meat.

Meanwhile, back at the office, you should be packing your own lunch anyway. If you have to spend lunch in a conference room, bring that brown bag and eat what's in it instead of ordering out with the rest of the group. Or if you do order out, nothing says that you have to get the big sub sandwich with salami and mayo. You should know better and order a turkey sandwich with mustard.

Don't beat yourself up. If you miss a workout once in a while, remember that it's not the end of the world—or even the end of your workout routine. If this was a regular occurrence, you probably don't work out at lunch anyway. So if it's once in a while, just enjoy it. Have a meal on the company's dime and give yourself a day off. "Just resolve to stick with the workout tomorrow and you won't get sidetracked," says Dr. Pace.

Climb the corporate ladder. You don't want to look like you're roaming the floor lost and with nothing to do, so don't do multiple laps around your floor.

Instead, expand to other floors of your building. For this part of the workout, do a lap around your floor, then take the stairs up to the next floor, walk the circumference of that floor, then hit the stairs again for the floor above that. Do three to five floors, then come back down, taking the steps as fast as you can.

Step it up. Find an isolated stairwell and try this calf burner. Step up on a stair with your right foot, slowly raise your heel off the ground, then step up with your left foot, raising your left heel. Since you'll be walking on the balls of your feet, be sure to hold on to the railing for balance. Walk up one flight in this manner.

Make a conference call. If your work life revolves around a cubicle, seek out some privacy and exercise in an empty conference room. "Conference rooms make excellent exercise rooms," says Amberge. "There's plenty of room to maneuver, and they're usually empty at lunch."

For starters, do push-ups and crunches, as many as you can. You can also do lunges and squats. Or grab two chairs (the nonrolling variety, please), position them on either side of you, put your hands on the seats, legs straight out on the floor in front of you, and do dips.

Cooldown

Don't head straight back to work after your workout. Take a few minutes to recover and prepare yourself for the rest of the workday. Here are two steps that will help ease you back to your desk, refreshed and ready to go.

Hit the water. If you've been doing these exercises at a brisk pace, you should actually feel a little winded. Don't park yourself at your desk just yet. Walk slowly to the water cooler. Fill your glass, drink it down. Have another. "It's always a good idea to rehydrate after any exercise," says Amberge.

Refuel. Now, to eat. Pick a spot a good 5- or 10-minute walk away and stroll over. Or if you brown-bagged it and weather permits, take your lunch and walk out to a nearby park. "The point is to do some slow, easy exercise that allows your heart rate to come down gradually, rather than abruptly stopping," Amberge says.

Office Stretching

Three Minutes to a New You

It's one of those days. You hit the snooze button on the alarm clock, but your just-five-more-minutes-please turns into 45 minutes. You jump into the shower, which alternates from scalding hot to ice cold as your wife does the breakfast dishes in the kitchen sink. You get dressed and rush downstairs, grabbing a cup of coffee that you promptly spill on your shirt and tie. Back upstairs for a quick change, then it's out the door with another cup of coffee for the road.

You slap a Janis Joplin cassette into the car stereo, which proceeds to chew it up right as Joplin is pleading for a Mercedes-Benz. As you futilely try to extract the tape from the voracious machine, you switch to the radio just in time to hear that a jack-knifed tractor trailer has caused a two-mile backup on the southbound lanes. Of course, you didn't really need the radio reporter to tell you that—as evidenced by the squealing of your tires as you slam on the brakes.

An hour later, you finally get clear of the accident scene and arrive at work late. You check your voice mail and learn that your boss left a message last night saying that he wanted the Henderson report first thing in the morning—which was now more than an hour ago. And the damn thing isn't even finished yet.

By now, your shoulder and neck muscles are so tense that they feel like they're going to snap. You frantically pound out the rest of the report and rush upstairs to hand-deliver it, only to be informed by the boss's secretary that he's out of the office at meetings all day but left word that he'd review the Henderson report tomorrow.

You resist the almost overwhelming urge to throttle her, smiling painfully, and head to the break room to grab your fifth cup of coffee of the morning. Like *that* will help calm you down. Here's a better idea. In less time than it takes for a coffee break—three minutes—you can enjoy a tension-relieving, flexibility-enhancing stretch break designed by Bob Anderson, author of *Stretching at Your Computer or Desk* and *Stretching* and co-author of *Getting in Shape*. For each, breathe easily and naturally and, as always, no bouncing. And you don't have to relegate these stretches to work—they're perfect for when you're in bed and just waking up or during a warm bath or shower.

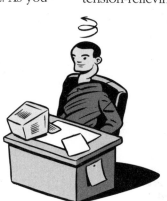

Shoulder Shrugs

Sit or stand with your arms hanging loosely at your sides. Shrug your shoulders up. Hold five seconds. Relax your shoulders downward. Do two or three times.

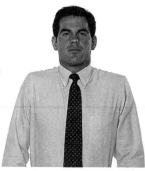

Neck Rotations

Sit or stand with your arms hanging loosely at your sides. Turn your head to one side, then the other. Hold for five seconds on each side. Repeat one to three times.

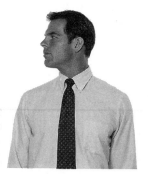

Arm and Shoulder Stretch

Lean your head sideways toward your right shoulder. With your right hand, gently pull your left arm down and across behind your back. Hold for 10 seconds. Repeat for other arm.

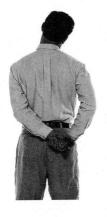

Chest Stretch

Place your hands shoulder height on either side of a doorway. Your chest and head should be up, your knees slightly bent. Move your upper body forward until you feel a comfortable stretch. Hold for 15 seconds. Do once. Do not hold your breath.

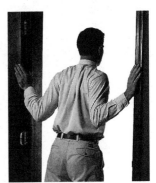

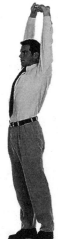

Shoulder and Wrist Stretch

Interlace your fingers above your head, palms up. Push your arms slightly back and up. Hold the stretch 10 to 20 seconds. Do twice. Do not hold your breath.

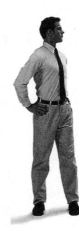

Trunk Rotations

Stand with your hands on your waist. Gently twist your torso until you feel a stretch. Hold 10 to 15 seconds. Repeat on the other side. Keep your knees slightly flexed. Breathe.

Quad Stretch

Stand two steps away from a wall and place your left hand on the wall for support. Standing straight, grab the top of your left foot with your right hand. Pull your heel toward your butt. Hold 10 to 20 seconds. Repeat for other leg.

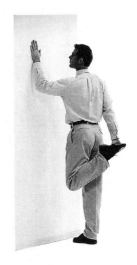

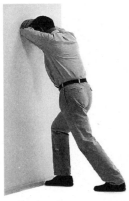

Calf Stretch

Stand slightly away from a wall and lean on it with your forearms, head resting on your hands. Place your right foot in front of you, leg bent, left leg straight behind. Slowly move your hips forward until you feel a stretch in the calf of your left leg. Keep your left heel flat and your toes pointed straight ahead. Hold an easy stretch for 10 to 20 seconds. Repeat for other leg.

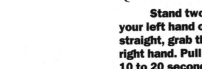

Office Exercises

Working Out While You Work

Researchers at Tufts University measured daylong energy expenditures among men and came to the conclusion that—you might want to hold on to your hats here, fellas—active guys were significantly leaner.

Whew, thanks for clearing that up. Actually, though, there was something truly surprising about their findings, because the kinds of activity the lean and mean crowd engaged in were not necessarily traditional exercise. Such unstrenuous exertions as shifting in your chair, pacing around your office, and even getting excited about a good idea add up to more calories burned, in the course of 16 waking hours, than a half-hour of sweating at the gym, the studies determined.

In other words, the little things do indeed add up. Or, as Susan Roberts, Ph.D., chief of the Energy Metabolism Laboratory at the Jean Mayer U.S. Department of Agriculture Human Nutrition Research Center on Aging at Tufts University in Boston puts it, "Whatever you do all day, do it vigorously."

Call Weighting

Okay, you say, how about all the time I spend on the phone each day? How do I do *that* vigorously?

We're so glad you asked. It's estimated that the average executive spends 15 minutes a day on hold listening to such mind-numbing fare as "Feelings" and the collected hits of Bread. No wonder the boss is always in a rotten mood. But there's no reason that you have to put ex-

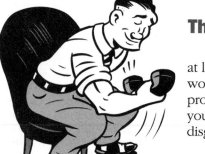

ercise on hold while you're waiting. Here are some ways to build strength without dropping the phone.

Squeeze, please. One of the first things you learned as a man is the importance of a firm handshake. So why not work on it while you're on the phone? Squeeze a therapeutic exercise ball, available at drugstores, for about a second, then release. Work up to 60 a hand.

Squeeze, and smile slyly. Another of the first things you learned as a man is the intense pleasure of orgasms. (Hopefully, that was a separate lesson from the one regarding firm handgrips.) For more intense orgasms, do 10 slow reps tightening and releasing your pubococcygeal muscles—the muscles you clench to stop the flow of urine. But concentrate on the exercise, not the erotic advantage you'll gain from it. There's no telling when that vice-president will come back on the line.

Do some curls. No, you don't need dumbbells on your desk. Just some rubber exercise tubing available at sporting-goods stores. Stand on one end with your right foot, and grab the free end with your right hand. Curl your hand palm up toward your armpit. Do 10 reps, then repeat with your left arm. Do three sets.

Take a stand. To build beefy calves, stand and hook your right foot behind your left ankle. Holding on to a desk for support, rise on your toes, then slowly lower. Do 30 reps, then repeat lifting your right heel.

The Office Gym

Odds are that you spend at least 40 hours a week at work. But in all that time you probably never realized that your office is actually a gym in disguise.

Okay, maybe not. But it does have possibilities.

"People ask me all the

time, 'How do I keep in shape at the office?' " says Joseph Barredo, a personal trainer at the elite Vertical Club in New York City, a gym that caters largely to white-collar workers in midtown Manhattan. "Many people think that they need a gym because they sit behind a desk for 10 to 12 hours a day. But a desk, copy machine, or even your briefcase can be used to get some decent exercise while you're at the office."

To prove his point, Barredo devised a routine of nine exercises that requires nothing more than two books or reams of copy paper, an office chair, a desk, and a briefcase.

"The ideal is to try to do this routine four times a week, but three times weekly should give you visible and felt results over a period of time," Barredo says.

Barredo recommends a minimum of 12 reps, and a maximum of 20 reps, for three sets of each of the following exercises, unless otherwise specified.

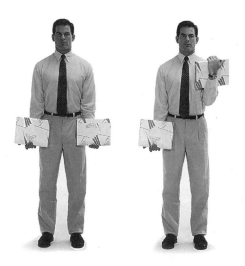

Biceps
Biceps Curls

Hold a book or a ream of packaged copy paper in each hand. With your feet slightly apart and knees unlocked, stand straight so that your shoulders are back and your upper torso is upright. Place your hands at your sides with your palms facing forward.

Bending your elbow, slowly curl your left hand up toward your left bicep, keeping your upper arm straight. Your wrist should be locked, and your palms should continue to face forward. Slowly lower your arm, and then repeat with your right arm.

Deltoids
Lateral Raises

Hold the books or reams of paper while you stand straight with your feet slightly apart and knees unlocked. Place your hands at your sides with palms facing your body.

Slowly raise both arms outward, as though you were flapping wings, keeping your elbows slightly bent and making sure that your thumbs are higher than your pinkies as you lift. Bring both arms up to shoulder height, and then slowly bring them back toward your sides. If you can't keep your wrists straight as you lift your arms, you should substitute lighter books or paper that can be lifted without bending at the wrist.

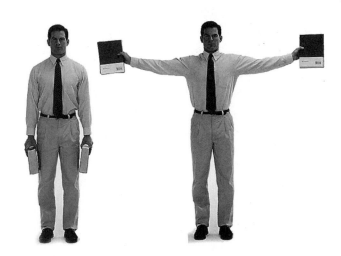

Triceps
Triceps Extensions

Sit in your office chair with your back straight and feet flat on the floor. Holding two reams of copy paper between your hands, place both arms straight up over your head.

Slowly lower both arms backward, bending at the elbows so that the paper touches your shoulders. Your palms should be facing the sides of your head. Then raise your arms slowly so that they are in the starting position.

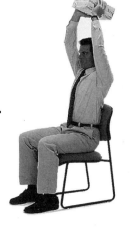
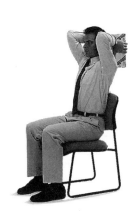

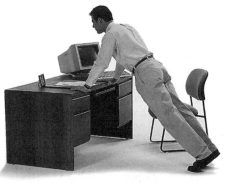

Triceps
Chest Press

With your hands shoulder-width apart and palms facing down, lean forward against the edge of your desk. Your legs and back should form a straight line, and you should be up on the balls of your feet. Your arms should be slightly bent, elbows unlocked.

Press down against the desk, with elbows bent and facing outward. Then press back up to starting position.

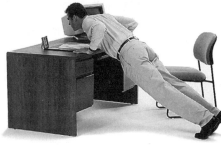

Quadriceps
Leg Extensions

Sit on the edge of a chair, with your knees slightly bent and legs together. Place your briefcase or a big book on top of your shins, bending your feet upward so that it doesn't fall off. Stabilize yourself by holding the sides of your chair with your hands.

Slowly lift your ankles to raise your legs upward. Don't lock your knees at full extension, but keep them at a slight bend. Your toes should be pointing up and out at a 45-degree angle. Hold the extension for two or three seconds, then slowly lower your legs.

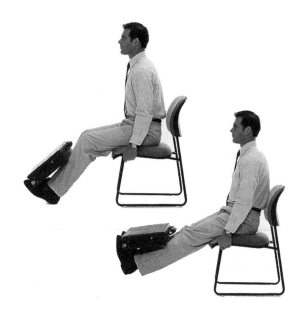

Adductor (Inner Thigh) Muscles
Adductor Resistance

Sit comfortably in a chair with your back straight, knees bent, and feet flat on the floor. Place your hands on your inner thighs, just above the knee joint. Pull your hands outward while you move your knees together. Hold for six seconds. Repeat five times.

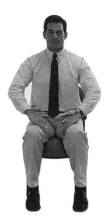

Abductor (Outer Thigh) Muscles
Abductor Resistance

Sit comfortably in a chair with your back straight, knees bent, and feet flat on the floor. Place your hands on your outer thighs, just above the knee joint. Press your hands together while you move your knees apart. Hold for six seconds. Repeat five times.

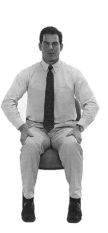

Obliques
Briefcase Side Bends

Stand upright with your briefcase in your right hand, palm facing in. Your feet should be shoulder-width apart.

Bend to your right, allowing the briefcase to drop down your right leg until you feel your obliques working. Keep your body facing front in the same plane—don't turn your torso into the side bend. Once you've gone as low as possible, return to the starting position. Do 20 reps. Then move your briefcase to your left hand and do 20 reps on that side.

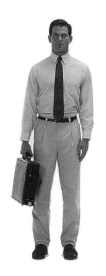
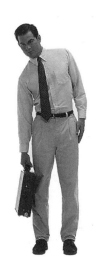

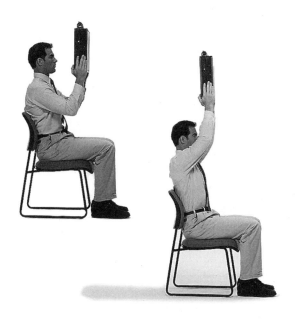

Deltoids, Trapezius
Shoulder Press

Sit comfortably in a chair with your back straight, knees bent, and feet flat on the floor. Hold your briefcase by the bottom corners with your palms facing inward, and lift it directly in front of your face with your elbows bent and in at your sides.

Slowly press the briefcase straight up toward the ceiling until your arms are fully extended above your head. Then lower the briefcase back to the starting position in front of your face.

The After-Work Workout

Powering Up
As the Sun Goes Down

As the hour hand on the office wall clock lazily approaches five, you're at an important period in your daily existence, and not just because you're about to be set free from the servitude of work for another day. No, the fact is that you're smack in the middle of the prime time of physical performance. You don't believe us? Just ask your body.

"We call it the power hour. It's a key point in your biological rhythms where many of the systems in your body that govern physical performance are operating at peak efficiency," says Dr. Phyllis Zee of Northwestern University Medical School.

According to Dr. Zee, studies show that our body rhythms change so that we reach a peak level of physical performance late in the day. It's why a lot of elite athletes like to work out and compete in the late afternoon and early evening. Our senses seem keener, our grip is stronger, and our muscle tone is better. We're able to tap an athletic potential that is often unavailable at other times of the day.

The reasons why aren't clear. Some experts have theorized that our late-day comeback hearkens to primitive times. Back then, when the sun was heavy in the sky, the theory goes, it was time for our forebears to quickly and sharply scan the terrain for shelter or food, before night descended and we went hungry, or worse, took on a new career as dinner.

Dr. Zee says that it's simply

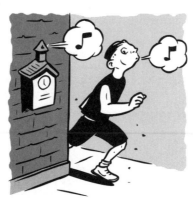

part of the rising and falling cycle of modern man's rhythms. Either way, when the day dwindles, our power increases. And what better way to expend that power than with a good workout?

When Work Is Over

As it happens, there are plenty of other less physiological reasons to work out in the evening. "First, it's a great stress reliever after a hard day's work. A lot of guys look forward to exercise as their reward at the end of a hard day, not as more work," says John Amberge of the Sports Training Institute. Also, he points out, exercising then makes for a good transition from work to home life.

"You have a chance to sort through the day and start thinking about what's going on at home, before you're in the thick of it," he says.

Tapping your late-afternoon power won't require a lot of preparation—just a little forethought. Try these tips and you'll see what we mean.

Have an after-school snack. Ah, the halcyon days of youth: The bus would drop you off at 3:30 or 4:00 P.M., and you'd march right into the kitchen for a snack. Even though your idea of homework has changed since school, you'd do well to pick up the after-school snack habit again.

"If you plan to work out in the evening, late afternoon is a good time to eat a little something—a cup of yogurt, a couple of bananas, a handful of pretzels. You'll have a little bit of fuel to help you through the workout. That way you won't be starving by the time dinner rolls around," Amberge says.

Change at work. When the whistle blows, break out your exercise togs before you begin your evening commute home. "I really recommend changing in your office or the bathroom at work. Then, whether you're going to the club or planning to work out when you get home, you can jump out of the car and be ready to go," says Amberge.

Cross paths with the club. If you're planning to join a fitness club, join one that's on your route to and from work. If you or your company already has a membership at a local club, try to plan your drive home so that you go right by the place.

"Especially in cities, a lot of clubs have a number of different locations. If it's too far off your usual route, you'll never go to it. But if you drive right by the place, you'll be hard-pressed to find an excuse not to go. I mean, it's right on the way," says Amberge.

Keep it light after dark. If you're planning to do serious weight training, confine it to the early evening hours. "Generally, you want to avoid really rigorous activity within two to three hours of bedtime," Dr. Zee says.

Adopting an exercise curfew will keep your body clock on the right track and ensure a proper night's sleep. "Body temperature and our sleep cycles are very closely linked," Dr. Zee explains. "At night, our temperatures usually drop slightly. But if you exercise hard right before bed, you can actually raise your body temperature, and that will keep you awake." By the time evening rolls around the next day, you won't have any energy for a workout.

Mix fitness with family. Amberge says that one of the reasons many men blow off working out at night is not because of fatigue but because of family. "You only have so many hours in the evening to see the kids, to spend quality time with your family," he says. And of course, your family's a priority, so exercise gets relegated to the back burner.

So combine the two. "You and your wife can work out, go running, cycling, whatever, together," says Amberge. "There's nothing that says that exercising together can't be quality time."

Warm up with the kids. Another variation of the family workout scenario is exercising with your kids. "First, of course, you get in some quality time; you're doing something with your kids. Second, you're raising healthier children in the process because you're showing by example how important exercise is to you," says Amberge.

Completing an Evening Circuit

No matter what time of day you work out, your routine should always have components of light and heavy exercise: the warm-up, the exercise routine, the cooldown, and stretching. Evening is no exception.

"If you've been sitting around all day or you've just been in a car or on a train for an hour, you'll definitely need a warm-up," Amberge says. "And a cooldown phase is just as important. The last thing you want to do at night is go through some heavy exercise and then collapse onto the couch or into bed. It's just too stressful on your body. You end up sabotaging all the physical gains you've been trying to achieve."

If you exercise at a club, you should always allow yourself 10 minutes of warming up with an aerobic exercise—rowing, stair-climbing, whatever you like—before hitting the weights. Then be sure to do 10 minutes of cooldown before you head home—a walk on the treadmill, perhaps, followed by some stretching.

Like many men, though, your workout is probably closer to home, and odds are that your basement doesn't feature the latest aerobic gizmos. In which case, incorporate the following basic elements into your evening routine. They'll ensure that your body is adequately prepared for whatever you throw at it—and help guarantee a good night's sleep.

Take a hike. Consider this part of your warm-up and also a good transition from work life to home life. Since you already changed at work, you're ready to go right out of the car. So go. Get out of the car and walk. Don't check the mail, and don't set foot in the house, unless it's to yell to the family that you're walking and they can come, too. Do two or three quick loops around the block, briskly walking, suggests Amberge.

Sprint indoors. Once you set foot back on your own property, move double-quick. Sprint up the driveway, dash into the house. Run to your wife, sweep her into your arms for

Fighting the Force of Darkness

It's dark when you get up in the morning. And it's dark when you leave work to come home at night. It's winter—the time when workouts go into the deep freeze.

"Sunlight—or the lack of it—can definitely have a detrimental effect on your resolve to exercise regularly," says Kirk Fisher, who should know. He's the fitness director for the Alaska Athletic Club in Anchorage.

"If we're lucky, we might get some light around 10:00 or 10:30 in the morning. Then, sunset's around 2:00 or 3:00 in the afternoon," he says. And yet, the Alaska Athletic Club is packed during the winter months, and Fisher works hard to keep his clients from straying back to their dens for a long winter's nap. Here are his strategies for sticking to a workout even when the forces of darkness are arrayed against you. If they work in Alaska, they'll work where you are, too.

Vary your workout. Every year when you turn back the clock, make a point of altering your workout routine completely on the same day.

"Throw in some completely new exercises; pitch a couple old ones that you didn't like," says Fisher. "So many guys get stuck in the rut of doing the same old exercises every day. Well, when it's time to turn back the clocks, you know it's time to mix up your workout. That sudden variety in your routine can often be all you need to stick with a program."

Look on the bright side. If you exercise in the basement, make sure that you keep the place well-lit. "Just bringing a couple of extra lamps down to the basement can really make a difference," Fisher says. "If it's dark and murky down there, you're just not going to exercise that much."

Get out. You might find it even more effective to leave your house and head for the bright lights of a fitness club. "We're packed during the dark months for a lot of reasons. One, the place is very bright—lots of light and mirrors. Two, there are other people here, and that in itself can be a motivator," says Fisher.

That's why he recommends hitting your local club or YMCA regularly in the winter. "You don't have to buy a full membership to go. We have a lot of people who just come in the winter and pay a guest or drop-in fee each time they go. It's not too expensive," he says. Call the clubs in your area for pricing.

Go toward the light. Lots of times, the thought of exercising when it's dark out is just too depressing, says Fisher. "So I suggest making a habit of doing some little bit of exercise when it's light out." Go for a walk at lunch; take a mid-morning stretching break. "The point is to do something active while it's light out. That may give you enough of a boost so that you can do your regular workout in the evening," he says.

a brief, powerful embrace, then run to your exercise equipment. If your workout of choice is an outdoor activity like running, then head back out the door. "Now your serious training work can begin," Amberge says.

Sit down for supper. After your main workout, refuel with dinner. "Most Americans make dinner their heaviest meal of the day, which is a mistake," Amberge says. The reason is that bedtime is only a few hours off, and research has shown that food eaten shortly before bed not only tends to keep you awake but also has a greater tendency to be stored as fat.

"The best thing about an evening workout is that, after exercise, you probably won't feel like throwing down a heavy meal," Amberge says. You'll more likely make more sensible choices, especially if you had a snack before the workout.

Take an after-supper stroll. Even if your appetite got the better of you, you can still minimize the damage by doing another few laps around the neighborhood. "Consider this a bit of a cooldown. Take it slow; you're winding down before bed," says Amberge.

What's for Dinner?

You've finished work and your workout. Now it's dinnertime. You've certainly earned a good meal, but you don't want to do anything at this point that will undercut all the good you've done for your body today. So to make the most of your exercise gains, here's a course-by-course listing of foods to embrace or avoid in the evening recommended by Georgia Kostas, R.D., director of nutrition at the Cooper Aerobics Center at the Cooper Clinic in Dallas.

• Soups. Avoid the heavy, creamy, or cheese-based soups. Stick with vegetable soups, bean soups, and tomato- and broth-based soups. They'll help you replace fluids and carbohydrates you lost while exercising.

• Salads. Fresh vegetables—especially tomatoes, dark green lettuce, spinach, carrots, broccoli, and beans—will add essential vitamins, minerals, and carbohydrates to your diet. For dressings, stick with something like heart-healthy olive oil (but go lightly!) and vinegar rather than those glutinous dressings.

• Meats. Although you might think that you owe yourself a nice juicy steak after a workout, you're better off eating a heavy piece of meat like that at lunch. Have a lean piece of chicken or turkey. On second thought, have a steak—a salmon or tuna steak or other seafood. You'll fill up without feeling too heavy. Other good choices in the seafood department include shellfish like steamed shrimp, crab, clams, and mussels, which not only are packed with muscle-friendly protein but also boast valuable nutrients like vitamin B_{12}.

• Pastas and grains. Yes, pastas are good after a workout—their complex carbohydrates make ideal fuel for your body. If you're planning to eat something like lasagna, stick with a small serving or a half-order, since the cheese and meat add extra protein and fat. Or opt for lighter grain dishes like rice, quinoa, or couscous (an African grain that's tasty and quick to fix). All are high in carbohydrates and low in sodium and fat.

If you choose pasta, avoid heavy cream sauces and even hot spicy tomato sauces—these may cause your stomach to "work overtime," which may keep you from getting a good night's sleep and may affect your performance tomorrow. Instead, try a marinara (meat-free) sauce made with basil, and add just a little bit of olive oil and a shake or two of Parmesan cheese.

• Vegetables. You can hardly go wrong in this category, as long as your choices aren't soaked in butter, cheese, or cream sauces. Rely heavily on vegetables like broccoli and spinach as well as beans. Eat steamed or stir-fried vegetables, never deep-fried vegetables. Eat salads with light dressings.

• Dessert. Fruit or low-fat yogurt (which contains protein and bone-strengthening calcium) is great. If you need something sweet, have a few spoonfuls of frozen yogurt, a couple low-fat cookies, or some low-fat hot cocoa.

On the Road

Tips for the Traveling Man

Wall-to-wall cardiovascular equipment. Tons of free weights. Stair-climbers, treadmills, and exercise bicycles delivered by room service. Gatorade stocked next to the imported beer in the mini-bar.

Workout heaven, you say? Not quite. Try the next hotel you'll visit.

It used to be that when you went out of town on business or vacation, you'd also say good-bye to your workout. If the plane, car ride, eating on the run, or nonstop meetings didn't derail your exercise plans, the hotel's "workout room"—often a closet with little more than a broken-down stationary bike—would.

But increased competition for your lodging dollars has led a growing number of hotels—from fancy resorts to more modest accommodations—to provide state-of-the-art fitness equipment and programs. Of the 45,000 hotels and motels in the United States, nearly half now have some gym or fitness equipment available to guests, says Marni Dacy, communications specialist for the American Hotel and Motel Association, the industry's largest trade association, in Washington, D.C.

As a result, if you pick the right place or simply just plan ahead, there's no reason—aside from some serious slacking off—why you can't keep your workout program on track. "Fitness amenities are just something that the consumer expects to have when he travels today, and the hotels that want to stay competitive are delivering," says Judy Singer, Ed.D., co-owner of Health Fitness Dynamics, a fitness and health spa consulting company based in Pompano Beach,

Florida, that has helped design or open more than 50 such facilities.

Fit to Travel

If you're like most of us, you're worried about losing all your hard-earned fitness while traveling. Unfortunately, your fears are not completely unfounded if you are a weight lifter.

Consider one study that involved folks in their sixties who worked out for four months straight and then took 10 weeks off. After the full 10-week break, the cardiovascular exercise group lost little in fitness. The weight lifters in the study, however, saw much more dramatic changes in their fitness levels. Within 5 weeks, resistance trainers showed significant strength losses. And by 10 weeks, they were almost back to where they started before beginning the four-month program.

But those who lost their fitness were able to recapture it and even improve once they returned to the gym. Both groups—the cardiovascular trainers and the resistance trainers—achieved higher levels of fitness when they hit the gym for another four-month program, according to Gary A. Storzo, Ph.D., associate professor of exercise and sports sciences at Ithaca College in New York.

Because working out on the road is fraught with logistical potholes that can impede your fitness progress, consider these tips the next time you intend to travel.

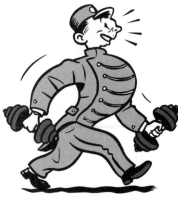

Make fitness a factor. When making your business or vacation travel arrangements, ask your travel agent to give you the lowdown on the fitness facilities available in hotels in that city, and make that a factor in your decision, says Dr. Singer.

Order the special meal. Virtually every airline worth its wings will provide a low-fat or vegetarian meal during flights if you order yours when you make ticket reservations, says Brenda Lucom-McKinstry, a United Airlines flight attendant who routinely travels by air four days a week and author of *Fitness on the Run*. (The book comes with two rubber exercise tubes. For information, call 1-800-FLY-1FIT.)

Pack a healthy snack. Since eating on the road is like playing Russian roulette with a fork, always have a healthy treat on hand like a cup of yogurt, fruit, or nuts and raisins, Lucom-McKinstry says. The same goes for journeys by car that are notorious for taking you past beckoning fast-food signs. "I find that poor eating habits compound travel fatigue," Lucom-McKinstry says. "I don't leave my house unless I have a Powerbar, some Fig Newtons, or something like that with me."

Take a walk. Trapped in layover purgatory? Rather than getting upset, get rid of your stress, burn some calories, and energize yourself by walking a few times around the terminal, says Dr. Singer. One swing through Atlanta's Hartsfield International Airport or Chicago's O'Hare can rack up several miles. Add the energy that it takes to dodge unruly luggage carts and travel-weary passengers and we're talking serious caloric burn.

Shell out for fitness. No doubt about it, exercise pays off. But you may have to pay a little extra for it. It's not often that you'll find exercise equipment in a budget motel (priced around $40 a night or below), says Dr. Singer. So you may have to pay a few dollars more for a hotel with equipment, but it's worth it.

Pack a bag. If you have to travel on a budget, you can do the next best thing: Bring your own exercise equipment. There's no need to rent a U-Haul for your Olympic bars and plates, though. From rubber exercise tubing to jump ropes and exercise tapes, carry-along fitness gear comes in all kinds of portable shapes and sizes, says Dr. Singer.

Consider cross-training. Are you a runner trapped in a hotel with a downtown that looks like war-torn Bosnia? Give the hotel's stationary bike or Universal weight-training machine a try. Are you a gym rat? Swim in the pool. Just don't try to train with reckless abandon. Your muscles and cardiovascular system are used to a different kind of workout, warns fitness consultant Dr. Adele Pace.

Check with the front desk. You forgot your gear and your hotel doesn't have an exercise room or equipment. Why settle for several days of self-imposed atrophy? There's a good chance that your hotel offers a free visit to a nearby gym or, at the very least, a jogging or walking map, says Dr. Singer. Ask the concierge or someone at the front desk for help. And don't forget to tip.

Turn on the tube. Instead of watching a bad in-room movie, click on ESPN, ESPN2, the Health Channel, or the Madison Square Garden Network. Many cable channels air exercise shows every weekday morning that provide not only good cardiovascular workouts but also fitness tips that can help you train better.

Try the old standards. Push-ups, squats, lunges, calf raises, crunches, and assorted other exercises need only your body weight and motivation to deliver a great workout when events and elements conspire against you, says Bob Lefavi, Ph.D., a sports nutrition and strength-training specialist at Armstrong Atlantic State University in Savannah, Georgia, and the 1990 International Federation of Bodybuilding North American bantamweight bodybuilding champion. "My wife thinks I'm crazy, but I've turned many a hotel room into a mini-gym doing these kinds of exercises," Dr. Lefavi says. For more information on weightless workouts, see The Core Weightless Workout on page 40.

Go to the well. It's not exactly scenic, but running or walking the hotel stairs can provide a tremendous cardiovascular workout if the weather is threatening or you're in an unsafe neighborhood, Dr. Singer says.

Stay an extra day. When planning to attend an out-of-town business conference, consider tacking a day or two on the beginning or end for a short fitness holiday. "Regretfully, the era of the two-week vacation has passed by many of us, but these mini-vacations are a great way to recharge your batteries," Dr. Singer says.

When Work Is a Workout

Getting the Most from On-the-Job Training

The pedometer on his belt tells the story. On a typical workday, United Parcel Service driver Don Spohn walks nearly 12 miles. You might expect as much from the lean, tanned 43-year-old Coplay, Pennsylvania, resident—Spohn was a cross-country and track star in high school. It's just that, back then, he wasn't hauling all kinds of heavy boxes and cartons with him.

On one of his former delivery routes, Spohn recalls, "I'd pick up 6,000 pounds of bearings in one stop. I'd pull out of there, and the back of the truck would practically be dragging on the ground."

Like many men across the country, Spohn's job is one heck of a workout. And with a daily regimen of after-hours strength training, he's been able to stay healthy. But statistics show a definite downside to strenuous jobs. The national rates for cumulative trauma disorders—injuries that most often affect workers' hands as they perform the routine functions of their jobs—have soared, increasing by nearly 1,000 percent in a recent 10-year period.

"In some warehouses, people are expected to lift a total of 20,000 pounds a day," says David Rempel, M.D., associate professor of medicine at the University of California, San Francisco, School of Medicine. "They're doing it in awkward postures, under stress, and at rapid rate. And if you don't do it quickly enough, your salary is reduced. Or vice versa: There are incentives for working very fast—all of which creates a risk for muscular and skeletal injuries to the shoulders and spine."

Some companies, automobile manufacturers among them, have redesigned jobs so that workers aren't carrying heavy weights as far or as often. Others have restructured assignments so that employees who perform repetitive tasks that can lead to injury—like sorting mail or typing—can take frequent breaks. Still, most companies that demand heavy or repetitive labor have a long way to go, Dr. Rempel says.

Fit to Work

While the research isn't overwhelming—only a few small studies suggest that fit workers are less likely to get injured on the job—physical therapists insist that greater aerobic capacity, flexibility, and strength can all help keep workers healthy.

"Most of the men who do these jobs don't look at what they do as being as physically taxing on their bodies as something like wrestling or boxing, but I'd say that it is," says Marge Rodgers of Genesis Rehabilitation Services. "Yet they wouldn't deny that the wrestler or boxer needs to train and to prepare for each bout. My job is not only to help them get better but also to stay in the fight longer without injury. Otherwise, they might as well just keep my card, because they're going to need to see me again."

Since getting in shape could mean the difference between a long, productive career or chronic pain—and employer-generated solutions could be years down the road—consider these tips for improving your job-related fitness.

Take frequent breaks. And we're not talking about the

coffee-related kind. Suppose you use a jackhammer day in and day out. Every 15 to 20 minutes, bend backward (not at the knees); straighten your arms, hands, and fingers; and reposition your feet. If you're typing at a computer or twisting a screwdriver, gently stretch your hands and wrists backward with your opposite hand. Plumbers scrunched under a kitchen sink should crawl out and lie flat on the floor.

"If you do that several times throughout the day, you probably won't use up five minutes in 8 hours, but you'll be cutting your risk for injury significantly. Maintaining normal motion in joints and muscles requires that we put them through their normal motion 5 to 10 times within a 24-hour period," Rodgers says.

Get aerobicized. Since most heavy labor tends to be anaerobic in nature, your postwork workouts should tilt toward the cardiovascular, says Rodgers. "It takes a bit more time, but even a 10-minute session of walking or riding a bike is better than none. Of course, 30 minutes or more is best for improving your cardiovascular system, and that's what many laborers need."

Find balance. Your chest, shoulders, and biceps look like they've been carved out of stone—no doubt a tribute to those eight-hour days hanging plasterboard. But did you know that neglecting your back could actually set you up for shoulder problems?

"Any time your chest is overdeveloped, the middle of the back—your rhomboids, lower trapezius, and the rotator cuff group as a whole—can become weakened and stretched," Rodgers says. The next time you're in the gym, skip the bench presses and train your back with several sets of lat pull-downs and a variety of rowing movements.

Stay hydrated. If the average person is supposed to drink eight glasses of water a day, where does that put a construction worker doing his thing in 93°F heat and 90 percent humidity? "The requirement wouldn't necessarily double, but it would make sense to drink that and several more glasses after work just to make sure that you're getting enough," Rodgers says.

Fall off the lunch wagon. Hot dogs, sweet rolls, candy bars, and sodas may be typical lunch wagon fare, but that doesn't mean that you have to climb on. "You don't see a lot of fresh fruits, vegetables, and salads on those things," Rodgers says. "But as far as I'm concerned, nutrition plays a big role in all of this. The nutrients have to be there for the body to handle the stresses the best it can."

Ask for help. You're probably rugged enough to tough out any work-related task on your own, but it makes no sense to put your health at risk, says Dr. Rempel. "One of the delivery companies recently raised its weight limit on packages from 75 to 150 pounds. The good news is that they've encouraged their drivers to ask for help when they have to deliver packages that heavy. We need to see more of that, and guys need to take advantage of it," Dr. Rempel says.

Say hello to dolly. Whether it's a dolly, winch, or a homemade version of a wheelbarrow, you can save yourself a lot of stress and strain using assistance devices, Dr. Rempel says. "These are low-cost ways of moving heavy materials that don't require constant lifting," he says. "You see a lot of creative ways of moving materials. Many of these ways are developed by workers themselves."

Wear a lifting belt. Although research shows no real benefit among workers who wear a lifting belt, there is some evidence that it may remind them to ask for help or use lifting assists when they move heavy objects, says Dr. Rempel.

Look critically at your career. Don't know how to train after work because you use so many different muscles during the day? Share your story with a personal trainer, and let him help you develop an exercise program that strives for balance, says Rebecca Gorrell, a certified exercise leader and wellness education director at Canyon Ranch Fitness Resort in Tucson, Arizona. An average session will cost you about $40—far less than a day without pay.

Staying Healthy on the Swing Shift

Don't Let the Clock Punch You

Anyone who has worked the swing shift knows what a grind it can be. Merely maintaining your health becomes a daunting task, and finding the time and energy to exercise is even tougher. That's the dilemma facing some 20 million American shift workers—from emergency services personnel and overnight delivery workers to clerical staff and computer programmers.

For one thing, few restaurants—other than the proverbial doughnut shop—are open when these folks are on the job, often limiting their food choices to glazed, jelly-filled, or chocolate-covered. Then there's the stress of managing family relationships, trying to get adequate sleep, and staying awake and alert while on the job. How about accidents to and from work? In one study, 32 percent of shift workers reported having an accident driving home from work in the past year.

In fact, shift work–related mishaps alone cost an estimated $70 billion annually in lost productivity, lost wages, medical expenses, property damage, and insurance costs, says Lynne Lamberg, author of *Bodyrhythms: Chronobiology and Peak Performance* and *The American Medical Association Guide to Better Sleep.*

The toll on workers' health is also high. Two-thirds of shift workers complain of disrupted sleep; twice as many

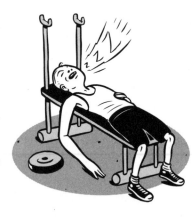

shift workers as regular folks develop gastrointestinal problems such as ulcers, diarrhea, or constipation—symptoms derisively called graveyard gut. Half of all shift workers smoke—twice that of the national average. And after five years on the job, shift workers are twice as likely to suffer heart attacks and heart disease as day workers of the same age and sex, Lamberg says.

"There's really no other conclusion here that you can draw. The human body is not designed to work through the night. Most of us are what's called diurnal—programmed to be awake and alert during the day," says Jack Connolly, Ph.D., president of ShiftWork Consultants, a consulting firm based in Springfield, Missouri, that provides support services to 24-hour operations.

Avoiding Occupational Hazards

All economic trends point to an increase in the use of shift workers—with some guys actually volunteering for duty, albeit reluctantly. "Rather than bringing on extra workers, employers are just making the people they have work longer," says Timothy H. Monk, Ph.D., professor of psychiatry and director of the Human Chronobiology Program at the University of Pittsburgh. "And in an environment where real wages are falling, people are taking on second and third jobs to maintain their standard of living. By definition, the second job is usually a shift-working job."

But whether you're new to shift work or an old pro, experts say that there are several practical things you can do to maintain a healthy lifestyle while working odd hours. Here's what they suggest.

Ease in a regular workout. For people who sleep at night, Lamberg says, physical performance is best around 5:00 P.M. Reflexes are faster, and coordination is smoother then. For people who sleep in the daytime, particularly those who frequently change schedules, the optimal performance time is harder to predict. The best time to work out, Lamberg says, is whenever it's most convenient. Having a special time is not as important as making time to do it. But if you can fit exercise into a regular time slot in your daily schedule, she says—right before or after work, for example—that's a plus. It will help keep your body clock in line and should improve your sleep, mood, and overall fitness.

Take your treadmill with you. During a visit to the control room of an electrical power company, Dr. Connolly observed that the shift workers had installed a rowing machine. "It looked like they would be able to exercise without ever being too far away from where they needed to be," Dr. Connolly says.

Go into morning. Those who punch out at around 7:00 A.M. should try to eat breakfast with the family, then read the paper and relax—literally puttering around the house for an hour or two before going to bed, says Lamberg. "The main thing is to try to get on a schedule and keep it so that your body can adapt as much as possible."

Go gentle into that good night. Guys who get off at 11:00 P.M. should probably forsake lengthy after-hours socializing—not to mention booze—and opt to hit the sack instead.

"There's a real temptation, particularly among police officers, to get together, chew the fat, and have a few beers," says Mike Bahrke, Ph.D., director of development for FitForce, a Champaign, Illinois, company that helps develop fitness programs and standards for law-enforcement agencies.

Other shift workers simply use alcohol as a sleep aid. In one small study, 32 percent of the shift workers reported using alcohol to fall asleep after their 12-hour day shifts, while 20 percent used it to sleep after their night shifts. It's far better, says Dr. Joanne Curran-Celentano of the University of New Hampshire, to eat a healthful meal containing complex carbohydrates—a bowl of cereal, for example—than to depend on alcohol to encourage sleep.

Cut the caffeine. And you thought the cast of *Friends* sucked down a lot of coffee? The typical shift worker drinks between seven and eight cups of joe a day—twice the national average.

"Obviously, they're trying to keep themselves awake, but too much caffeine has well-known negative effects on the cardiovascular system. It increases resting heart rate and blood pressure, and it can create arrhythmias in people with tendencies toward irregular heartbeats," says Dr. Connolly.

Not only that, but caffeine stays in your bloodstream for five hours, disrupting sleep patterns, Dr. Monk warns. His recommendation: If you're on the night shift, don't take any caffeine after about 4:00 A.M. If you're on the evening shift, avoid it.

Put some light on the subject. Instead of having the boss pay for another industrial-size bag of coffee, ask him to spring for brighter lights, which studies show may help keep shift workers more alert, Lamberg says.

Lay down the law. Social taboos prevent us from calling anyone at 2:00 A.M. unless it's an emergency. So why aren't shift workers spared afternoon calls—for some, their prime sleeping time? Often it's because family and friends haven't taken their sleeping schedule seriously. Make sure that people understand that calls and other interruptions aren't appreciated. Point out that you'd probably be more fun to talk to after some rest anyway, Dr. Monk says.

Nap if you need it. Since evening shift workers actually report better sleep than those who work 9:00 A.M. to 5:00 P.M., they probably won't need a nap. But studies show that those who work the night shift may benefit from a two-hour afternoon nap, says Dr. Monk. "We're not talking about 10 to 20 minutes here. The research shows that you'd need a much longer nap to see any benefit," he says.

Making Exercise a Family Affair

Show That You're Fit to Be a Father

Mission accomplished. You snuck out of the house for a Saturday morning run while your kid was glued to the tube, and you set a personal best before the end of the Bugs Bunny hour. But now that you're back and your endorphins are flowing, it's time to switch off the set and use that energy to build some more exercise into both of your lives.

"A recent study found that the more TV a child watches, the more likely the child is to be overweight, both because it promotes inactivity and because the advertising encourages them to make poor food choices," says Mary Ann Hill, director of communications for the President's Council on Physical Fitness and Sports in Washington, D.C.

In fact, federal research shows that 4.7 million U.S. youths between the ages of 6 and 17 are severely overweight. That's 11 percent of children in that age group and more than twice the rate of the 1960s, says Hill.

Family Matters

Increased TV watching isn't the only problem. Video games, the Internet, unsafe neighborhoods, and the elimination of many physical education classes—while effectively stamping out those ill-fitting blue gym shorts—have all combined to make kids even pudgier and less active.

Of course, wishing Mortal Kombat had never been invented won't make it go away. And if both you and your wife work, the challenge seems doubly daunting. But by trying at least once a week to make exercise a family affair, you'll send several messages: Your kids and wife are important to you, good health matters, and Sebastian Cabot is gone but not forgotten. Heck, you'll probably even burn a few calories.

"It's important for families to be active together and establish that habit," Hill says. "You'll be nurturing the innate love of activity that children have and giving them many more opportunities to be active while adding some natural activity into your day. And you'll probably find that it's lots of fun."

Here are some suggestions to get you started.

Put a sharp pencil to it. You plan business meetings, vacations, even dental appointments for Pete's sake. Why should making sure that your family is getting enough exercise be any different?

"Things that you want to include in your week have to have a time and routine," says Judith C. Young, Ph.D., executive director of the National Association for Sport and Physical Education (NASPE) in Reston, Virginia. "Some families have a family game night. Some commit to spending Saturday out and about together. The trick is being faithful in not allowing other things to interfere with that time." For more ideas, the NASPE also publishes a brochure called 99 Tips for Family Fitness Fun. To request your free copy, write to 99 Tips, c/o MET-Rx Foundation for Health Enhancement, 2112 Business Center Drive, Irvine, CA 92715-1014.

Trade cookies for a game of catch. A warm, well-timed chocolate chip cookie says "attaboy" like few other treats known to man—or child. But when a kid does something great, the reward doesn't have to be fattening. In fact, it can be downright healthy, like a trip to a batting cage or miniature golf. Or just go out in the backyard and play catch. "It's another way of saying that doing something physically active can be even more rewarding than consuming things," Dr. Young says.

Milk that milk run. Need a gallon? Got a grocery store within walking distance? Take a walk together. Your children can ask you the tough questions, like whether electricity had been invented when you were a boy. "It's not as much of a workout as you could hope to get at a gym, but at least it's better for you than just driving your car to the store." More time to come up with answers, too.

Rake and roll. You have a snowblower with enough horsepower to clear a mile-wide path before most folks can say "The Weather Channel." But getting the kids involved in leaf and snow removal is a good way to keep them active and create family yard fun.

"You can say, 'As soon as we get this cleaned up, we can build our snowman or snow fort or jump in the leaves,' " suggests Dr. Young. And if you let them jump in the leaves, you can start raking them up again—hence burning more calories and making your kids really happy.

Pick your own. Okay, even the most shopping-challenged dad could find the produce section of the local supermarket and arrive at the checkout lane with the ingredients for a decent salad. But would that make him a healthy dad?

You can turn nutritious shopping into a fun-filled, fat-burning event by visiting a farm where you pick your own fruit or vegetables. "It's not heavy labor and the kids will probably do more running around than picking, but it's a great way to get everyone physical and together as a family," says Dr. Young.

Doing the Sporting Thing

What do you do when you have children who are interested in a variety of sports, but you don't have much time or energy at the end of a workday to spend with them?

Kevin McManus, a 40-year-old feature writer for *The Washington Post* and father of eight-year-old Johnny, created what he and his little guy call a Major Sports Day.

First, they gather up the gear: a soccer ball, a basketball, tennis balls, a bat—sometimes even a Frisbee. Then they head to the child's former nursery school about a half-mile from their home in Silver Spring, Maryland.

For the next two to three hours, the pair moves from sport to sport. McManus pitches while his son swings a bat. During soccer, they alternate as attacker and goalie. When they take the basketball court, Johnny shoots an undersized ball at a regulation hoop while dad rebounds and feeds it back to him. And so on. And as McManus points out, there's "no scorekeeping, no drills. Just repetition of a few basic moves.... It's emotionally fulfilling for me to see how much pleasure it gives him to do all this stuff," he says.

Master thespianism. Instead of letting your kids be brainwashed by another mindless video, why not read to them and let them act out the story? Or let them practice their reading while you perform, says Dr. Young. You don't need spotlights to see each other sweat. Who knows, you might discover a child prodigy or launch your own acting career.

Get in the Olympic spirit. Forget the gold medals and sappy feature stories. The next time you have a neighborhood block party or family picnic, make sure that someone organizes several athletic events that both kids and adults can play together. One quick way to spoil the fun is to take yourself and the competition too seriously.

Being a Social Guy

Meeting Friends and Lovers at the Gym

The thumping bass lines of blaring dance music aren't all that discos and fitness clubs have in common. Back in the *Saturday Night Fever* days of the 1970s, discos were where you went to see and be seen, to make friends, and—perchance—to meet women. Oh, and you could work up a pretty good sweat working out on the dance floor. Today, you can do all that and more at most health clubs.

"It's become such a social milieu for so many people that at peak hours there are lines to use the machines in gyms across the country," says Courtney Barroll, a certified personal trainer and medical exercise specialist at Equinox Fitness Club in New York City. "These are people who want to stay in shape, but they also want to get to know people. The great thing is that they can do both."

What is it about exercise that brings out the social animal in many of us? Maybe the same thing that makes any successful relationship possible: common interests. And for a busy guy with no time to network, read sappy personal ads, or join a dating service, working out may be one of the best ways to find friendship and even *amore*.

"Whether you're talking about romance or friendship, you can't build a relationship with someone if you don't enjoy doing things together," says Marilyn Fithian, Ph.D., co-director of the Center for Marital and Sexual Studies in Long Beach, California. "Exercise,

sports, and outdoor activities all provide a good starting point for these opportunities."

Training Partners

Positive relationships help give your immune system a boost and reduce the effects of stress, dislocation, or isolation you may feel at work, research shows—not to mention a myriad of other health benefits. And working out together may even help rekindle a flagging marriage or romance. Here are some tips that should help spice up your workout life.

Go slow. A shapely young lass wearing form-fitting workout gear asks you how to use the Smith Press Station, also known as the Smith machine. You're single, flattered—and proceed to wax eloquent on its versatility, safe construction, and quad-blasting capabilities. She smiles; you swoon. Easy, Buster. Don't jump to any conclusions . . . yet. "Gyms are a relatively safe place. Most women don't think that anyone who is likely to do them harm is going to a gym and working out. But just because some woman talks to you doesn't mean that she's interested in something. It's my guess that most women feel safer there than they would in a bar, for example, and, as a result, are probably friendlier," Dr. Fithian says.

Pop the question. If you don't mind looking or feeling a bit awkward, consider asking her how to use a piece of equipment or how she trains a particular body part. You can also comment on an article that you're reading while you work out or changes at the gym—whatever it takes to get the conversation started. Just make sure that she's warming up or cooling down.

"If she's running hard or in the middle of a set, don't approach her," Barroll says. "Let her get her workout in or she might be annoyed."

Let loose with some lingo. It's typical for early discussions to focus on reps, hiking routes, or 10-K times and not much else. This kind of chitchat helps establish similarity—a vital part of successful relationships, says Howard Ruppel, Jr., Ph.D., executive director of the American Association of Sex Educators, Counselors, and Therapists in Mount Vernon, Iowa.

Fall back on the familiar. "You may not know what to talk about, but if you're involved in some kind of activity like tennis or an aerobics class, you can always talk about that," Dr. Fithian says.

Know when to fold them. If you decide that she is not interested or doesn't know how to respond, you can simply smile and proceed to the next machine. If she does something similar, *don't* follow. "You've shown her the interest. Now the ball is in her court," says Barroll.

Offer her a bite. If you're getting good vibes and would like more, ask her out for a protein drink, post-race carbofest, or just a cup of coffee. "You can tell a lot from a brief interview," Dr. Fithian says. "One cup of coffee or whatever doesn't mean that you're committed to a lasting relationship. You can always walk away."

Prime the pump. If you're already in a relationship, does your partner feel neglected when you ride with the boys? Take time to take her for a spin before you hit the hills. Leaving her behind may make her less interested in sex later. Studies show that exercise boosts levels of HDL (high-density lipoprotein)—the so-called good—cholesterol, which, in turn, can influence sexual desire, Dr. Fithian says. So exercising with your partner may be as good for your sex life as it is for her health. Talk about a win-win situation.

"If you're an avid cyclist, spend 15 to 20 minutes of your ride with her, and then you can go with your friends," says Dr. Fithian. In a study of 173 triathletes, those who reported the best relationships talked about training's impact and worked out as often together as possible.

Alone Again, Naturally

With the assistance of Courtney Barroll of Equinox Fitness Club, we've determined some of the most annoying habits and behaviors men exhibit while working out. Incorporating these into your workout won't make you popular with the ladies, but it will keep the machines near you free.

Grunt with gusto. "This is the number one complaint that I hear," Barroll says. "The average woman who wants to keep in shape in a club environment is extremely annoyed by men who grunt. It's a big turnoff. They always ask, 'Why do they have to make all that noise?' And you know something? I never really know what to tell them."

Make like Barney. "Straining is not attractive, and neither is turning purple," Barroll says. "Plus, it's dangerous."

Slip on some spandex. "Most women like traditional baggy boxers and big T-shirts. They think that those are much cuter," Barroll says. "Tight T-shirts and shorts leave nothing to the imagination."

Be a condescending know-it-all. "Some women might welcome advice, but others take offense. And sometimes it's too late before you figure out just where she stands," Barroll says.

Reveal your rhythmic impairment. "Tripping during an aerobics class has nothing to do with being sexy," says Barroll.

Brandish your back hair. "It doesn't get much worse than this," says Barroll.

Weekend Workouts

Building a Better Body— And Home

It's been a great week, workout-wise. Even though it was busier than usual at the office, you managed to get to the gym or head out for a run every day. Now, it's the weekend.

And life really gets hectic. The list of errands and chores on your refrigerator is as long as *War and Peace*. Grocery shopping. The Farmer's Market. Mowing the grass. Chopping firewood. Running the kids to soccer practice. And you wonder: When am I going to find time to work out?

Relax. Those weekend chores that you view as insurmountable obstacles to exercise just might provide a better workout than your normal routine at the gym. And if they don't now, they can—with a little bit of planning.

A Chore Thing

Look at the numbers: An hour of digging or intense snow shoveling can burn more than 700 calories—about the same as running. Chopping wood is good for more than 400 calories, nearly as much as skating or skiing, and hauling firewood can torch more than 900 calories per hour. Even painting, carpentry, weeding, and mowing the lawn boost your heart rate to bona fide "aerobic" levels.

"We have to start looking at our homes less as fitness enemies," says Bryant Stamford, Ph.D., director of the Health Promotion and Wellness Center at the University of Louisville

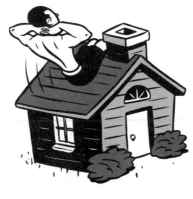

and author of *Fitness without Exercise.* "They present us with countless opportunities for exercise that we tend to view as annoyances. Whether it's a clogged toilet, a hole in the roof, shutters that need paint, or a rain gutter that backs up, it's exercise—a calorie burner, a step toward a healthier heart. Your lawn, your leaves, and your soiled home can save you. Calories burned at home count just as much as those burned at the gym."

In some cases, they could count even more.

"There are plenty of data that show that 30 to 45 minutes a day, done year-round, of many types of physical activities will reduce the risk of heart attack—and that includes some of what you consider weekend chores," says Arthur Leon, M.D., an epidemiologist and cardiologist at the University of Minnesota in Minneapolis who has studied the effects that leisure activities have on the risk of coronary heart disease. "But things like heavy weeding, gardening, digging, and mowing the lawn are all really moderately hard work and also improve flexibility because of all the bending over you have to do."

"There's also a mental boost to doing weekend chores," adds Dean Johnson, host of the long-running PBS home-improvement series *Hometime.* "Sometimes when you're not in the mood to do something around the house, the realization that you're also accomplishing some exercise by chopping wood or doing whatever can really help. You're doing something good for your body as well as your home."

While few argue that weekend chores can help improve health by reducing the risk of heart attack, some experts question how much they can improve overall fitness—especially in guys who are already in good shape.

"If you're sedentary, then any physical exertion that you do will help," says Dr. Barry

Franklin of William Beaumont Hospital Rehabilitation and Health Center. "But if you're already fit and a regular exerciser, then mowing the lawn, gardening, or doing home repairs will offer little additional cardiorespiratory activity to improve your aerobic fitness level."

Unless, of course, you make it tougher than it has to be. Here's how.

Do it like Grandpa. "Probably the most obvious thing that you can do to get the best workout doing chores around the house is to do them the old-fashioned way," says John Emmett, Ph.D., associate professor of physical education at Eastern Illinois University in Charleston. "That means using a push mower instead of a gas-powered one, a hand drill instead of a power drill, and a snow shovel instead of a snowblower." Keep in mind that a warm-up is always a good idea before beginning any vigorous activity.

Studies on snow shoveling show that using a shovel burns 42 percent more calories than spending the same amount of time clearing your walk with a snowblower. "Basically, it's a question of just walking with a snowblower versus doing some really intense exercise," Dr. Emmett says. He estimates that with other chores, you can burn from 10 to 40 percent more calories using "low-tech" manual tools instead of ones powered by gas or electricity.

Can the coffee breaks. "Any job where you are consistently moving, especially while climbing or lifting or carrying something, may help to improve health and fitness levels," says Dr. Franklin.

Pick up the pace. And the faster you move, the better. When mowing your lawn, for instance, Dr. Emmett suggests power walking behind a lawn mower (even a gas-powered one) for a better workout. "Although fast walking with a lawn mower may not result in a better cut, you can do what I did when I used to mow lawns working my way through college: Double-cut it by going over the same area at a 90-degree angle. That way, if you power walk, it'll take you about the same amount of time as a single cut, but it will result in a better job and you'll get a better workout."

Think big. Go for the biggest and heaviest tool you can get and you'll get a better workout. Besides, you'll likely finish your chores sooner.

"So use a 20-ounce hammer instead of a 16-ounce one for a better workout when you're nailing," says Dr. Emmett. "The same goes with using a big snow shovel instead of a smaller one. It will take less time to complete the job, and you'll get a better workout because it's more intense." Injuries, however, may be more likely, so be careful with heavier equipment, says Dr. Emmett.

Stretch beforehand. If you plan to build a deck on the weekend, make sure that you've been building your muscles during the week. "The thing that you *don't* want to do is be a weekend warrior who's in pain on Monday morning because you tackled a job without being in shape," Johnson cautions.

"Most home-improvement jobs won't exercise you aerobically as well as something like running, but they do require a lot of lifting and heavy moving—things that require good back muscles. If you tackle them cold, you could get hurt, so it's a good idea to work these muscles beforehand. I use a weight machine, but at the least, you should do some stretching before tackling anything that requires heavy lifting."

Switch hands. It may be awkward at first, but one way to make any job more taxing is to do it left-handed, assuming that you're normally a rightie. "Besides giving yourself a better aerobic workout (you use more energy working your 'weaker' side), it also helps build up muscles that you normally don't use as much," Dr. Emmett says.

While you won't want to do this when painting or using hand tools, Dr. Emmett says switching hands is a good way to increase intensity when chopping wood, shoveling snow, or performing other already-labor-intensive chores. To prevent injury, he suggests working the nondominant arm sparingly at first and then increasing its workload over time as it gets stronger.

Time-Saving Tips from the Pros

*Top Trainers Share
Workout Secrets*

Whether it's catching a jet for a sales trip or buying stock for a client just before the NASDAQ soars, seconds count in the business world.

But you don't have to leave that philosophy in the locker room when you hit the gym. Although there's never an excuse for sloppy exercise technique, there are dozens of safe ways to shave time from your workout routine—and still train like a champ. Here are some of the most effective, based on interviews with exercise professionals.

Practice some fancy footwork.
Simply changing your foot placement from exercise to exercise can turn a simple leg press into a total leg workout, says Courtney Barroll of Equinox Fitness Club.

Placing your feet as close together as you can without touching, for example, fires the center part of the quadriceps a little more. Placing your feet a little wider apart, about hip distance, and putting pressure on the outer part of the feet emphasize the lateral (outer) part of the quadriceps. Positioning your legs on the outer corners (toes on a slight angle out to take stress off your knees) also works your butt more.

Attack the opposites. Train opposing muscle groups during rest periods. For example, after you get done doing bench presses,

switch to seated rows for your upper and lower back. Just finished training your biceps curls? Do triceps extensions. "This is a really time-efficient workout that I do regularly," says Steven Wheelock, fitness co-director of Canyon Ranch Lifestyle Resort in Lenox, Massachusetts.

Stay focused. You've heard it before: He who fails to plan plans to fail. Add this corollary: He who walks into the gym and wanders around wastes massive amounts of time, according to Rebecca Gorrell of Canyon Ranch Fitness Resort. Plan your routine before you walk into the gym, and do your best to stick to it—unless circumstances or opportunities dictate otherwise.

"We ask our clients to focus on their fitness goals because they can be overwhelmed with all the choices or start talking to other people about fitness programs," Gorrell says.

Rev up your fat-burning furnace.
Treadmills are great for walking, jogging, or running, but doing a little of each by interval training can help kick your body's fat-burning ability into high gear, says Barroll. Start with 5 minutes of walking as a warm-up. Then jog for 3 minutes and run at a higher level for 2 minutes, alternating back and forth. Continue alternating until you reach the 30- to 40-minute mark and then allow yourself a 5-minute walk to cool down, Barroll says. "This routine always seems to go quickly, and it's a great fat burner," she says.

Be a Versa-tile guy. When it comes to hardcore cardiovascular workouts, it's hard to top the VersaClimber. That's because this machine forces you to use virtually every major muscle—and lots of smaller ones—as you push, pull, and climb your way to fitness, says Joe Ogilvie, a fitness leader at Chelsea Piers Sports and Entertainment Center in New York City. In fact, at least one research study showed that training on a VersaClimber required more oxygen use in

Trading Workout Places

In one of Dan Aykroyd's best movies, *Trading Places*, our hero portrays a buttoned-down business type who's cruelly yanked from the lap of luxury and dumped into the street to make way for a hustler played by Eddie Murphy. Now it's true that Aykroyd got to spend significant screen time with Jamie Lee Curtis, a plus in any guy's book. But that's not the main point here, gentlemen. It's how he adapted to his new surroundings and came out on top. Imagine a similar situation at your gym—your once comfortable and familiar surroundings now too crowded to allow you to follow your routine in order.

Rather than bag your workout, you can avoid the masses by simply trading exercises and equipment. Not only will you save time, but incorporating different movements will help force your muscles to grow. Consider the alternatives.

If you can't do this...	Do this...
Bench press	Flat bench dumbbell flies, presses, cable crossovers
Inclined bench press	Inclined dumbbell presses, dips (leaning in so that your chest is parallel with the floor)
Barbell rows	Cable rows, one-arm dumbbell rows, T-bar rows
Front lat pull-downs	Pull-ups, dumbbell pullovers
Overhead triceps extensions	Triceps kickbacks, overhead dumbbell extensions, cable triceps presses, dips
Barbell curls	Dumbbell cable curls, concentration curls
Seated military barbell press	Seated dumbbell press, alternating dumbbell press, standing dumbbell front raises
Upright barbell rows	Lateral raises, standing dumbbell front raises
Squats	Lunges, step-ups, leg presses
Crunches	High leg lifts, V-sits, knee-ups

college rowers than running on a treadmill and using a rowing machine.

"It's been my experience that most people get a tremendous workout even in as little as 10 minutes—the VersaClimber is very effective," Ogilvie says.

Bring a bottle. You could take a hike to the water fountain every time your mouth screams for a drink. A better idea, though, is to bring a plastic bottle filled with water, diluted juice, or sports drinks. And you won't just be saving time. Dehydration is also one of the main causes of cramping, which can really put a crimp in your exercise plans, explains Barroll.

Don't peak. If you want to train for peak performance, avoid training at peak hours—between 6:00 P.M. and 7:45 P.M. in most gyms. You'll wind up wasting time standing in line for machines. "It's really tough to get a good, concise workout then because it's usually so crowded," Barroll says.

Join the dawn patrol. Most gyms have fewer patrons in the early-morning hours. Not only that, but you'll often find that your fellow exercisers are less talkative—perhaps because they haven't gotten revved up for the day yet, Barroll says.

Bear down on a bench. A single

bench can be your workout island in a sea of exercise chaos, allowing you to do chest and shoulder presses, triceps extensions, upright rows, pullovers, and other exercises—even crunches. This workout goes smoothest when you have an array of barbells and dumbbells nearby but can be performed with either, according to Barroll. "The only time that you'll have to move is to grab different weights," Barroll says.

Warm up wisely. It makes sense to warm up by walking on a treadmill—just 5 to 10 minutes raises your body temperature, helps get the blood flowing, and lubricates your leg joints. But you can also help prepare for an upper-body workout by performing lateral and front arm raises and weightless shoulder presses while you walk, says Barroll. "Sometimes I'll do backward arm circles and then throw a few punches to break it up," Barroll says.

Take the cardio cross-train. If your gym enforces a 20-minute limit on all cardio machines, you can still get in a great workout simply by switching from treadmill to bike and rowing machine or stair-climber for 20 minutes each, Barroll says. "That way, you can get in a full hour of work and never leave the cardio area."

Cut socializing short. You look forward to chatting with your pals at the gym, but when time is short and you have to fly through a workout, tell them. That way, you can get your workout in—without making them feel like you're ignoring them. "One of the biggest complaints I hear is, 'I was there for an hour and a half, and I was talking for half of it,' " says Marc Goodman, a fitness instructor and personal trainer at Crunch, a gym in New York City.

Beat the clock. When you're crunched for time, try taking a 30-second rest between sets instead of a prolonged break, says Goodman. "Keep an eye on that second hand and then, boom, it's time for your next set," he says.

Train with your partner. Since exercise can seem like it's stealing time from you and your significant other, why not go to the gym together? And you don't have to actually move through the workout together either.

You should both understand that your training programs are probably very different, says Goodman. "It's better than feeling like time is being taken from each other," he says.

Major in "gymography." It may take some hunting, but you'll save all kinds of travel time if you can find a gym that is either on your route to work or on your way home, Goodman says.

Make a stash. A permanent locker at your gym containing extra shaving gear, soap, and maybe even an extra pair of shorts and shirt can help you when you need to train in a pinch, says Goodman. "It's worth the investment if your gym offers them," he says.

Go to prep school. You probably don't lay out your work clothes the night before, but prepping for your next exercise between sets can help save time. If you're going to use dumbbells, for example, pull them from the rack and place them at the bench you're going to use. If you're going from squats to leg presses, load the machine with plates. And so on. This also alerts others to your interest in the equipment, says Wheelock.

Gravitate toward a Gravitron. If you need to get in a good arm and back workout fast, this combination pull-up and dip machine can't be beat—unless of course you consider its unplugged cousin made by Cybex. Both machines are designed to provide enough assistance so that almost anyone—regardless of their fitness level—can do pull-ups, chin-ups, and dips at will, Ogilvie says.

Put yourself on the rack. Your gym buddies may not appreciate it, but you can cut training time dramatically by spending your time in front of the dumbbell rack instead of constantly moving from one machine to another. Consider the range of exercises within easy reach: shrugs, rows, inclined and flat bench presses, flies, curls of all kinds, shoulder presses, lateral raises, lunges, triceps extensions, and many others, says Ogilvie.

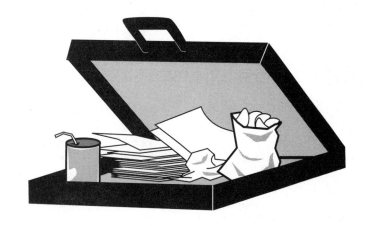

Part Four

Getting the Edge

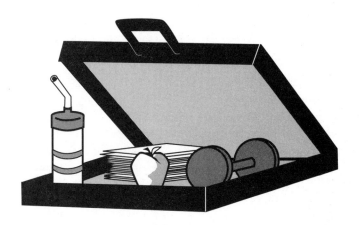

Packing a Lunch That Packs a Punch

Make It Fast, Nutritious, and Delicious

These days, your power lunch is more likely to consist of clocking a few miles along Main Street than knocking back a few martinis on Wall Street. But if you only have an hour or so to spend on the midday meal—and you're spending all of it working out—your lunchtime exercise may be one in futility.

"You need to eat a good lunch if you want to make the most of your workout," says Nancy Clark, R.D., director of nutrition services at Sportsmedicine Brookline in Massachusetts and author of *Nancy Clark's Sports Nutrition Guidebook* and two other books on eating for athletic performance. "You have a car, and you put gas in it, right? Well, you have a body and you need to put gas in it, too, if you expect it to run. Food is fuel for your body."

Remaking Your Muscles

Using the right fuel can mean the difference between getting a lot of mileage from your workouts every time you hit the road, weights, or basketball court, or breaking down quicker than Dad's old Rambler.

"Every time you work out, what you're actually doing is breaking down muscle and connective tissue, and when they rebuild, hopefully they come back stronger than before," says Pat O. Daily, M.D., director of cardiovascular surgery at Sharp

Medical Center in San Diego and chief executive officer of Daily's Fit and Fresh Restaurants, a chain of eateries serving low-fat, healthy foods. "What you are doing with food is replacing those losses in tissues."

But *how* you rebuild those muscles depends on what you eat—and when. Scarf down a steady regimen of lunchtime Big Macs (or other fat-laden foods) and that's what you'll become: big, Mac. And we're not talking about your biceps, triceps, or delts. Fat doesn't feed your muscles, just your love handles.

"Although fat is a nutrient we use as a fuel source, in most cases, the average guy stores about 75,000 calories worth of fat in his body, so it's not a nutrient that he's in short supply of—even if he exercises at lunch," says Kristine Clark, R.D., Ph.D., director of sports nutrition at Pennsylvania State University's Center for Sports Medicine in University Park. "Besides, fat is the slowest nutrient to be digested, absorbed, and metabolized, so while it may not adversely affect athletic performance, it certainly doesn't help it."

Eating for Power

So what does help? Foods rich in two important nutrients—protein, whose main purpose is to help build (and rebuild) muscle tissues broken down during exercise, and complex carbohydrates, the main "fuel" for energy. The average man's diet is 35 percent fat, 45 percent carbohydrate, and 20 percent protein. While most guys get enough protein, the problem is that it's often in the form of high-fat foods like meats and dairy products.

But many guys—especially active ones—fall short in complex carbohydrates, which are found in bread, cereals, rice and other grains, as well as plant foods like bananas, potatoes, and corn. Nutritionists recommend upping your complex carbohydrate intake to about 60 percent, while whittling down the fat in your diet to about 20 percent.

So what you want is a lunch that's easy to prepare and quick to eat (since you'll be spending most of your lunch hour exercising). Here's what the experts recommend for a brown-bag lunch that's quick to prepare and eat and nutritious enough to keep your lunchtime workouts in the pink.

Take a fresh look at carbohydrates. Mention carbohydrates "and everyone thinks of starchy foods like breads, bagels, cereals, and pasta," Dr. Clark says. "But carbohydrates actually come in four food groups—dairy, fruits, vegetables, and the starchy grains. What I recommend for guys who are working out at lunch is that about an hour or two before they exercise, they eat carbohydrate-rich foods in the fruit or dairy categories—or even better, combine them, like having a banana or other fruit and low-fat yogurt."

One advantage to these foods is that they tend to be lighter than the starchy carbohydrates; they're also easier to eat in an office setting than a plate of pasta. "Even though fruit and yogurt have relatively small amounts of fluid, they are very important for guys who work out. Even a 2 percent level of dehydration can impair athletic performance," Dr. Clark adds. "Besides, what could be easier to bring to work? Yogurt is ready to eat and can be left unrefrigerated for a couple of hours before you eat it. And all you need to do is peel a banana or other fruit."

Get right with egg whites. Despite eggs' reputation for breaking more hearts than Don Juan, the only real problem is in its yolk center. An egg white may be the world's perfect food—containing a mere 17 calories with no fat or cholesterol, and a decent 3.5 grams of muscle-building protein. (By comparison, the yolk contains 59 calories, over 5 grams of fat, 213 milligrams of cholesterol, and only 2.8 grams of protein.)

"What I personally do for my lunch when I'm working out is hard-boil some eggs in the morning and eat three or four egg whites for lunch," Dr. Daily says. "Sometimes I crush them

up in a cup of yogurt and eat that for lunch."

Keep a bottle handy. Dr. Clark recommends keeping a 16-ounce bottle of your favorite liquid on your desk and trying to consume the entire bottle at least an hour before exercising. "You may feel that you're overdoing it, but you will feel better during your workout," she says.

Immediately after your workout, try to drink another 16 ounces to replenish lost fluids. "It doesn't matter what you drink, although carbonated fluids like soda might increase gastrointestinal discomfort. Juices are good because you're getting vitamins, but they contain a lot of calories. Even coffee and tea are okay, though their slight dehydrating effect might seem more noticeable during warmer months simply because we perspire more at that time." Her recommendation is plain old water.

Say cheese. While many cheeses are a high-fat source of protein, some are relatively low in fat and pack plenty of nutrients. "Feta and mozzarella are good choices, but there are now plenty of low-fat or fat-free cheeses that make for an easy and nutritious lunch," adds Dr. Clark.

Go fish. While meat is high in protein—and fat—most fish gives you the muscle-building protein you need without the added fat. "As long as it's prepared without adding any fat, most fish, except for salmon and shark, is relatively low in fat and packs plenty of protein," says Dr. Daily. "Albacore tuna packed in water is among the best choices." A three-ounce serving contains only 111 calories, with just a trace of fat, and packs a whopping 25 grams of protein; it also contains nearly an entire day's worth of vitamin B_{12} and is a good source of niacin and iron.

Shed the skin. Carnivore sandwich-lovers, take note: You can indulge your craving for a hearty lunch that won't stick to your gut, as long as you remove the skin. "Chicken breast and turkey are also excellent sources of protein and can be low-fat if you remove the skin," adds Dr. Daily.

All-Day Eating Strategies

Refueling for Extra Power

Yeah, yeah, regular exercise can help you avoid being one of the 171 poor saps who drops dead of a heart attack every hour. Sure, it can prevent scores of other diseases, boost energy, lower weight, improve your sex life, and even make you think more clearly.

There are a million reasons *why* we should exercise, but many of us Y chromosomers focus on just one: We work out so that we can pig out. An extra mile might translate to an extra slice of pizza, while another set on the tennis court might mean another helping of potato chips . . . without having to buy elastic-waistband pants.

But while how much we exercise can help determine how badly we can eat without paying the full price (read: love handles), what we eat—and when—also plays a role in how well we exercise.

Eating to Win

The right foods, eaten at the right time, can actually improve your athletic endeavors—making you stronger and able to last longer.

"When you're talking about nutrition for maximum athletic performance, you're really talking about three things—eating foods to give you enough energy to do your workout, eating foods to give you energy afterward, and getting enough fluids to keep

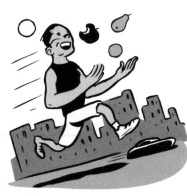

yourself hydrated so that you have energy for both," says Dr. Kristine Clark of Pennsylvania State University's Center for Sports Medicine. "Besides drinking plenty of water or other fluids, it means concentrating on low-fat, nutrient-dense foods both before and after exercise. In other words, carbohydrates."

That's because carbohydrates are the best food source for replacing glycogen, the main energy source that fuels our muscles for exercise. "When you exercise, you deplete your body's glycogen stores, and carbohydrates are the best way to replenish it so that you can go out and do it again the next day," says James J. Kenney, R.D., Ph.D., nutrition research specialist at the Pritikin Longevity Center in Santa Monica, California, and author of *The L.A. Diet*.

"Sure, if you're a professional football lineman, sumo wrestler, or Olympic heavyweight weight lifter and want to maximize your performance by adding bulk, eating a high-fat, high-protein diet might be advantageous—provided that you don't mind a life span that might be 20 years shorter than average. But for the rest of us, there are better ways to nourish yourself before and after exercise to get the most from your workout—no matter when you exercise."

Eating before Exercise

Of course, there's a wrong time to pig out on these right foods: immediately before you exercise. "It generally takes one to two hours for any food—even good ones—to be digested, absorbed, and metabolized to be utilized for energy," Dr. Clark says. So anything you eat within an hour of exercising just sits in your stomach.

And the more food sits in your belly, the worse your workout will be. Most experts advise against having a meal—600 calories or more—two to three hours before you start exercising. But that's not to say that you should go on a hunger strike to get a good workout. Just follow these experts' advice.

Remember the 60/60 rule. While pigging out before exercise can hurt performance, a little snack before it can actually help. Dr. Clark suggests the 60/60 rule—a light snack containing up to 60 grams of carbohydrates at least 60 minutes before your workout. (Guys who exercise first thing in the morning can eat it immediately before exercising, but their "real" breakfast should follow their workout.)

Among the snacks that fit the bill are five dried figs, two cups of grapes, a cup of low-fat yogurt, or a bagel and piece of fruit. Whatever you choose, just make sure that you eat it at least an hour before exercising, says Dr. Clark.

Forget the fiber ... for now. Eating high-fiber foods right before you exercise can lead to gastrointestinal discomfort and force you to interrupt your workout for a hurried and potentially embarrassing bathroom break. Neither option exactly enhances your workout, so nutrition experts recommend avoiding fiber power-houses such as high-fiber cereals before you hit the gym or the road. Although fruits, vegetables, and grains provide some fiber, they probably won't create any problems for you.

Eating after Exercise

A big drink is probably the first thing you need after any kind of decent workout. (Or maybe several drinks; Dr. Clark says that you need 16 ounces of fluid for every pound lost during exercise.) But fluid isn't the only thing. Here's how you should refuel your body with food after exercise.

Eat ASAP. You've heard of carbo-loading before exercise? Well, research shows that it may be just as important to carb out afterward, particularly if you exercise every day. "Even if you're a weekend warrior and playing a couple of hours of tennis on Saturday, if you

plan to play again on Sunday, you need to replenish your glycogen stores or else you'll fade out," Dr. Kenney says. "And research shows that the best time to do that is as soon after you finish exercising as possible."

For morning workouts, this translates to a postworkout breakfast of cereal, bagels, or other high-carbohydrate foods; for evening exercisers, pasta, bread, and beans are excellent choices, says Dr. Kenney.

Don't be a flour child. Now's the time to fiber up, so be sure that you're getting the most per mouthful. "Read the ingredients label of grain products, and if you see the word *flour* as the first ingredient, make sure that it's whole-wheat or other whole-grain flour," says Dr. Kenney. "White flour and other refined flours are not very nutritious compared to whole-wheat flours. Focus on whole-grain breads, pasta, and other grains that haven't been refined."

Veg out. Guys who work out to control their weight can get a helping hand—and extra helpings—if they load up on vegetables, especially for dinner. "Fruits are great, but vegetables have an edge because they tend to be more nutrient-dense and, on average, contain less than half the calories of fruits," says Dr. Kenney. "Three servings of fruit contain about 180 calories, while four servings of vegetables have only about 100 calories." That means that if you're the kind of guy who goes for quantity, you can *really* load up on vegetables.

Advice: If you're battling the bulge, start off each postworkout meal with a big salad. "Actually, instead of having a big bowl of pasta and a large serving of bread with a side salad, make the salad the main focus of your meal, with smaller portions of bread and pasta," says Nancy Clark of Sportsmedicine Brookline. That's because besides being high in carbohydrates—with about 40 grams per cup—pasta is also high in calories, with about 200 calories per cup (and few guys eat just one cup). But if you add an equal cup of beans to your salad, you'll get even more carbohydrates and fiber and fewer calories.

10 Great Preworkout Foods

Man doesn't live by pasta alone—or at least he shouldn't. While this low-fat, high-carbohydrate food has become as important to marathon runners and other endurance athletes as a tube of Ben-Gay once was, there are plenty of other low-fat, high-carbo-hydrate, workout-aiding foods that can boost your workouts and are more convenient. The following are among the best choices.

Bagels

"They're high in carbohydrates, low in fat, convenient, and delicious," says Evelyn Tribole, R.D., a nationally known nutritionist who wrote *Eating on the Run*. "What more could a guy ask for?" Not much, apparently, since a bagel (minus the fixings) has about 1.5 grams of fat, less than 200 calories, 31 grams of carbohydrates, and 6 grams of protein, which is needed to feed workout-weary muscles.

Bananas

Just peel and eat—no sticky juice or bothersome pits. What you do get is plenty of potassium, which can help head off leg cramps. "All fruit is good, but bananas are slightly higher in carbohydrates than many other fruits, and they're probably the easiest fruit to eat," says Tribole. Each banana has about 105 calories and more than 1 gram of protein, along with 27 grams of carbohydrates.

Broccoli

Former President George Bush hated it, but when was the last time you saw him shooting hoops after dark? Considered by some to be the single best vegetable there is, broccoli falls short in the carbohydrate department (only four grams), but a meager half-cup provides an entire

Wet Your Appetite for Exercise

The easiest way to prevent being a workout washout is to give your insides a good washout—with plenty of fluids.

"Studies show that even the slightest level of dehydra-tion, as little as 2 percent, can impair athletic performance," says Dr. Kristine Clark of Pennsylvania State University's Center for Sports Medicine.

And during a good sweat, you easily can lose that 2 percent—or more. Besides helping avoid dehydration, which can occur when you sweat, getting plenty of water also can prevent fatigue, cramps, pulled muscles, and other sports injuries, says Dr. James J. Kenney of the Pritikin Longevity Center. Here's how to make sure you're getting enough liquids.

Weigh yourself. "It's okay to lose one pound per hour of exercise (this is primarily glycogen and fluid deple-tion, which can easily be regained in a couple of hours after your workout). But if you weigh yourself before your workout and then again after it and see that you've lost three to four pounds, then you're not drinking enough fluids

day's worth of vitamin C, two grams of fiber, and two grams of protein. Plus, it can be eaten raw.

Carrots

And you wonder how Bugs Bunny still looks so great after all these years? Here's what's up, Doc. Each carrot has only 31 calories, more than 7 grams of carbohydrates, and 2.3 grams of fiber. Plus, it's the single best source of vitamin A you can find, which protects against cancer and can boost immunity (so you don't need to miss your workout because of illness). "For guys, I recommend the bags of baby carrots because they come already washed and taste great," Tribole says. Throw a few on your salad for added nutrition.

before, during, and after your exercise, and you're risking dehydration," says Dr. Kenney. *Advice:* Replace each lost pound with 16 ounces—or two big glasses.

Suck down some soup. While water is the best pre-workout and postworkout drink, it's not the only way to get your fluids. "Any liquid is fine, and that includes soup," says Dr. Clark.

Meanwhile, fruit juice is a good source of nutrients but has as many calories as soda, so don't guzzle that OJ. "And forget those sports drinks unless you're doing intense aerobic exercise for at least 90 minutes," says nutritionist Evelyn Tribole. "They're very expensive, high in calories, and don't really benefit the more casual exerciser."

Toast the morning. No matter when you exercise, you need to drink a glass or two of *something* first thing when you wake up. "Your body hasn't had any fluids for about eight hours, so it's very important to drink first thing when you wake up," says Nancy Clark of Sportsmedicine Brookline.

and you're getting a low-fat, high-carbohydrate food that's easy to eat and good for you," Tribole says.

Leftover Pizza

The breakfast of champions . . . or at least bachelors. But don't laugh. Pizza is high in carbohydrates and relatively low in fat if you don't slam it with pepperoni, sausage, or fat-laden cheeses, according to Tribole. Make it yourself with fat-free cheese and you'll save 3 grams of fat per slice. The crust contains B vitamins. Plus, each slice has 20 grams of carbohydrates and 7 grams of protein in 140 calories.

Sweet Potatoes

Packing nearly 28 grams of carbohydrates, 3½ grams of fiber, and 2 grams of protein, this 117-calorie tater is among the top choices for guys who hate to cook. Just stick a few holes in it with a fork and microwave it for a minute or so. "Besides, one sweet potato a day gives you all the beta-carotene you need," says Dr. Pat O. Daily of Sharp Medical Center and Daily's Fit and Fresh Restaurants.

Grape Nuts

"They contain more carbohydrates per bite than other cereals, and they're so dense," says Tribole. Stick them in the microwave for a great hot cereal (for those cold-morning runs). You can find cereals with more fiber, but that may be why Grape Nuts are a great preworkout snack.

Instant Beans

If you thought a cup of beans was only for hoboes, you haven't been shopping lately. These days, several manufacturers make "beans in a cup" that are microwaveable, nutritious, and cheap. "If you want a snack or meal on the run, they're great—just pop them in the microwave

Toaster Waffles

Frozen waffles can have less fat than homemade ones, with no irons to clean afterward. Plus, each heat-and-eat waffle has about 14 grams of carbohydrates and 2½ grams of protein. And because it's enriched, you'll even get a bit of bone-building calcium and some iron to boot. And what could be easier?

Yogurt

Hey, guys get osteoporosis, too—so hedge your bets with this high-calcium snack that makes for the perfect preworkout snack. Calories range depending on its fat content, but all yogurt is a good source of vitamin B_{12}, riboflavin, protein, and yes, carbohydrates.

Burning Off Fast-Food Calories

Don't Get Caught in the Speed Trap

The main appeal of fast food for busy guys is pretty obvious. It's fast. If you have an hour for lunch, you can cram in a 45-minute workout and still have time to hit the drive-thru lane at your favorite burger joint and make it back to your desk before the big hand strikes 12—or the big boss strikes you.

The problem is that, in a fraction of the time you spent exercising, you can easily pack on *three times* as many calories as you just burned—or more.

Find that hard to swallow? It's not—that's the problem.

To illustrate the point, we've put together a few scenarios that may sound familiar. (Not to you, personally, of course. But we're sure that you have a friend who has been in these kinds of situations.) We'll take a typical meal from a leading fast-food restaurant and provide examples of how much exercise a 180-pound man would need to burn off the calories. Then, we'll offer a suggestion of a healthier alternative from the menu that's just as fast but less fattening.

Breakfast

You jump out of bed for an early-morning appointment that could help make you salesguy of the month. After a quick shower, you put on your best suit, hop in the car, and zoom off. Mindful that eating breakfast helps boost your metabolism, you spot a Burger King and sail into the drive-thru. Within 30 seconds you bite into a warm sausage, egg, and cheese Croissan'wich. You arrive early at the meeting, close the deal, and celebrate by pumping iron for an hour at the gym.

Nutritional Cost

In the five minutes it took you to order, receive, and polish off that tasty breakfast sandwich, you packed on 600 calories and 46 grams of fat.

Workout Rx

Better head back to the gym. That hour you spent lifting weights only torched 342 calories. To burn off one little breakfast sandwich, you'd need to spend about an hour on the rowing machine (558 calories). If you'd rather shed the flab at home, surprise and impress your wife by scrubbing floors for an hour (522 calories) or washing windows for two hours (576 calories).

A Better Idea

Getting the same breakfast sandwich with ham instead of sausage will trim 250 calories and almost half the fat. Or you could head to McDonald's. Sure, you'll find plenty of high-fat offerings—a sausage biscuit with egg there has 520 calories and 35 fat grams. But some franchises sell fat-free apple bran muffins that are just 170 calories each. And if your taste buds are set on a breakfast sandwich, the Egg McMuffin packs a relatively modest 290 calories and 13 grams of fat.

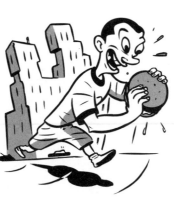

Lunch

It's one of those rare days when you understand what athletes mean when they talk about being "in the zone." You arrive at the golf club at 6:00

A.M. to play the front nine with the boss before work. After losing by a stroke (Gosh, how did you miss that putt on the ninth hole?), you're still in the office by 8:00 A.M. You write two memos that are models of clarity and conciseness. You defuse a couple of potentially explosive personnel situations with an aplomb that would leave most diplomats jealous. Now, you're heading out with the guys in the department for the all-you-can-eat buffet at the nearby Pizza Hut. No waiting for slow table service; just help yourself and chow down. You grab a plate, and six slices of Meat-Lover's Pan Pizza later ("Heh, heh," you chortle to your mates, "they sure lost money on me today"), you head back to the office bloated and sleepy.

Nutritional Cost

Each mouth-watering slice packs 340 calories and 18 grams of fat. Multiply by six slices and the grand total is a whopping 2,040 calories and 108 grams of fat.

Workout Rx

You should have limited your slices to the golf course. Sure, you walked off 617 calories playing golf. And that close loss was certainly good for your career. But if you want to pig out at Pizza Hut, you might want to take up a new sport: like trekking across the Arctic Tundra for 2½ hours on snowshoes. (Sorry, no huskies allowed.) If cold weather isn't for you, you could try scuba diving for three hours. Although after all you ate, you might just sink to the bottom like a stone.

A Better Idea

Even if you still downed six slices, by opting for Pizza Hut's Thin 'n' Crispy pizza with ham, you could have saved 936 calories and cut out more than half the fat.

Dinner

Some house-painting jobs are tougher than others. And this is one of them. That intricate woodwork looks great, but it's a pain to paint. You work up a man-size sweat on a muggy midsummer's afternoon, putting in three hours of tough labor before a thunderstorm rumbles in unexpectedly. Tired and sore, all you can think about is a long, cool shower and a good meal. Then you remember: There's nothing in the fridge! You spot Colonel Sanders's kindly visage looking down on you from a KFC sign on the next corner, pull in, and grab a bucket of Extra Tasty Crispy chicken to go. While watching a *Baywatch* rerun—and wondering how it's possible that the gifted Yasmine Bleeth hasn't won an Emmy—you down a couple breasts, a thigh, a cup of baked beans, potato salad, and cornbread. A well-balanced meal, no? No.

Nutritional Cost

We're in the bonus category again, pal. This meal set you back 1,958 calories and, worst of all, a stupefying 111 grams of fat.

Workout Rx

Those three hours of backbreaking work you put in this afternoon? Here's the balance sheet: calories burned—1,134; calories gained—1,958. That leaves an extra 824 calories you've packed on, much of it fat. You could head back out and do more manual labor—like, say, two hours and 10 minutes of hedge trimming—or you could jump rope for an hour and 12 minutes. But after an afternoon of hard work; a big, fat-laden meal; and an hour of *Baywatch*, odds are that you'll be dozing on the couch in no time.

A Better Idea

If you really need a chicken fix, KFC's Tender Roast provides a healthy alternative to their higher-fat fare. Two skinless breasts and a skinless thigh weigh in with a total of 444 calories and 14 fat grams. Substitute green beans (45 calories, 1.5 grams of fat) for baked beans, coleslaw (180 calories, 9 grams of fat) for potato salad, and a biscuit (180 calories, 10 grams of fat) for the cornbread and you wind up with 849 calories and 34.5 fat grams. Not great, but at least it gives you a shot at staying slim enough to be pulled ashore by Yasmine Bleeth if you ever find yourself caught in an undertow.

Packing the Perfect Gym Bag

How to Be a Quick-Change Artist

Socks. Sneakers. Jockstrap. Shorts. T-shirt. Towel. Maybe a clean pair of underwear if you can find one. Seems simple enough, right? So why do so many of us get it wrong?

"I can't tell you how many guys manage to forget something in their gym bags, and it ruins their entire workout," says Ken Karpinski, author of *The Winner's Style* and other books on the way men dress. "Just last week, I went to a tennis club with a friend of mine who realized when he was unpacking his gym bag that he forgot to bring socks. It took him about 25 minutes to get a pair. So much for our game."

Here's how to make sure that never happens to you (again).

Start at the bottom. One of the best ways to pack your bag is to do it from the bottom up. "Think of everything you need, starting at your feet and working up," Karpinski says. "Sneakers should go in the bottom, with socks inside your sneakers so you'll never forget them. Then shorts, a change of underwear, an athletic supporter if you use one, T-shirt or sweatshirt, and so on. You should pack in the reverse order of how you dress so that you'll spend as little time as possible looking for what you need. Besides, sneakers should go on the bottom of your bag to keep your clothes from getting dirty. Finally, don't forget any paraphernalia that you might need, such as weight-lifting gloves."

Other items that your gym bag should include are a toiletries kit (complete with talc, cologne, a comb or brush, soap, and deodorant) and a towel.

Make yours plastic. Some gym bags have separate pockets specifically designed to carry your smelly workout clothes after a workout. But if yours doesn't, Karpinski suggests also packing some plastic grocery bags. "This way, you can put your gym clothes right into the bag after your workout to keep them separated from everything else. It will keep your bag from getting too smelly."

Take a lesson from swimmers. A bath towel can take up to half your entire gym bag, and the more cramped your bag is, the more likely you are to forget to pack something. So take a lesson from Olympic swimmers and dry yourself off with a large chamois—a super-absorbent cloth often made of sheepskin. "It's as thin as the same kind of chamois you use on your car and absorbs 20 times its weight in water," says Karpinksi. "You can buy it in any good sporting goods store, and it's much better than a towel for your after-workout shower."

Concentrate on cotton blends. You might think that 100 percent cotton workout clothes are your best bet because they're so absorbent. "Actually, they can be *too* absorbent and may get heavy during an intense workout," Karpinksi says. "Very often, cotton blends—those made with some man-made fibers—are even better because they're also absorbent, without getting as heavy as all-cotton workout clothes."

Dressing for the Gym

Even if you put your body through the wringer with a work-place workout, your clothes don't have to look that way. By dressing right and storing clothes properly while you're exercising, you can keep business attire in the same top shape as what's underneath them.

Suits

A locker room can turn Armani into mush, especially after your workout when your freshly showered body can give your suit more wrinkles than an aging sun worshiper. Here's how to keep yourself looking crisp for the entire day.

Choose the right weight. Lightweight suits are just that when it comes to preventing wrinkles, so you're better off wearing one that's medium to average weight on workout days. "Look for a wool or wool-blend suit that's called a 10-month weight, or made from 10-ounce material," says Karpinski, whose other books include *Mistakes Men Make That Women Hate* and *Red Socks Don't Work.* "They have more body and resist wrinkling better. And the fabric breathes, so after a workout, you'll stay cooler, since the fabric allows some of the heat that builds up from both working out and showering afterward to dissipate a little."

Favor dark suits. "You shouldn't be worried about reflecting the sun's rays if you work indoors, but you should be worried about all that grime in the locker room," Karpinski says. "If you have a nice tan suit, the slightest dust or grime will show on the suit, and it'll be ruined for the day. But darker suits hide that dirt better."

Shirts

If you're a shirt-and-tie kind of guy, you know the importance of looking crisp—and staying comfortable. Cotton and cotton-blend shirts are your best bet on both counts, but they're more likely to wrinkle than man-made fibers. Here's how to dress without worrying about looking wilted—even if you are.

Don't hold the starch. Dress shirts should always be professionally laundered to keep them looking their best. And to keep *you* looking your best, ask for some starch.

"Heat and moisture coming off your body after a workout or shower will wilt a shirt, but having them lightly starched will prevent that and keep the shirt looking crisp," Karpinski says. "Medium starch is also okay, but the more starch you get, the quicker your shirts will wear out, so avoid heavy starch."

Be a button-down man. A button-down shirt is less likely to lose its shape in the collar than other types, and that's important for guys who hang their shirts on locker hooks. "And if you are hanging your shirt in a locker, use the locker loop on the inside of the collar," says Karpinski. "Just hanging it by the collar causes it to lose its shape more quickly."

Storing Your Clothes

A closet's hanging bar is the best way to hang onto your dress clothes, but you may not always find them in your corporate gym or health club locker room. "If there is place to hang your clothes with wooden hangers, that's great, because you can benefit from all the other guys taking showers and give your suit and shirt a quick steam," Karpinski says. But when hanging room is scarce, here's how to keep your work clothes looking great while you're out playing.

Use your car as a closet. "If you're driving to where you exercise, you should leave your suit jacket on a hanger in the backseat," says Karpinski. "Most locker rooms have reasonably small lockers anyway, and some don't have hanging bars." Even if they do, there's less chance for wrinkling in your car, and your wallet and other personal items are probably safer tucked under the seat.

Get looped. The best way to hang pants during a workout is either by their cuffs with a clamp hanger or folded over a wooden bar hanger. But if you're limited to a small locker, then hang your pants on a hook by a belt loop.

"Some guys like to hang their pants by the inside waistband, but that can create a puffy or wrinkled look over time," he adds.

Hit the Showers

Just Follow Your Nose

Thanks to the benevolence of your employer, you have exactly one hour for lunch. In those 60 minutes, you want to change into workout clothes, warm up, exercise, cool down, shower, dress, and maybe even eat lunch.

So it's obviously not the time to take a long, leisurely shower. But if you're going back to work, skipping a shower isn't a very pleasant option—especially for your co-workers.

If you don't know why, take a deep breath.

Working Up a Sweat

"Showering after a workout is a good idea, because if you're going to have any kind of decent workout, you're going to sweat," says Norman Levine, M.D., chief of dermatology at the University of Arizona College of Medicine in Tucson. "That's because sweating is the body's way of dissipating heat and keeping itself cool.

"In fact, in many cases one way to gauge the quality of your workout is how much you sweat. Well-conditioned athletes tend to sweat sooner and sweat more than people who aren't in as good shape. That's because their whole sweating apparatus is geared toward cooling themselves down. So if you're in decent shape, expect a decent sweat."

And unfortunately, an indecent odor.

There are two types of sweat: Eccrine is the odorless, colorless fluid that covers the entire body, the stuff that drips off the body. Meanwhile, apocrine is the nasty stuff—the thicker sweat in your underarms and groin area. Both are released when you exercise or do other activities that raise your body temperature, giving off a one-two punch that makes showering the perfect conclusion to a midday workout.

"The sweat from the apocrine glands has some odor itself, but the action of bacteria on apocrine sweat is what *really* gives the odor in your armpit and groin area," says William Dvorine, M.D., former chief of dermatology at St. Agnes Hospital in Baltimore. He also holds 11 black belts in various martial arts. But here's how to not sweat over sweating and make the most from your lunch-hour shower.

Lather up. While even the quickest lunch-hour rinse will remove sweat from your body, using soap regularly when you shower might allow you to occasionally skip some of those hurried cleanings. "Using an antibacterial soap kills the bacteria on the skin that can cause or contribute to body odor," says Dr. Dvorine.

So if you work yourself into a lather during your morning or evening shower, there's less bacteria on your skin come workout time, resulting in less chance of body odor, and hence less need for a midday shower. The good news is that nearly all commercially sold soaps have antibacterial qualities.

Take five before you revive yourself. If you take a shower while you're still sweating, expect to walk out of the locker room looking like you just came in from the rain. "That's because your body needs time to cool down after your workout," Dr. Levine says. "Otherwise, you're going to reactivate the sweating apparatus that's trying to cool down your body."

While there are no hard and fast rules about how long

you should wait—it depends on the outside temperature, the temperature of the shower water, and how much you've been sweating—Dr. Levine advises waiting until you start to feel yourself cooling down. "If you're hot when you jump into the shower, you might be hot when you get out of it. You should wait until you feel yourself start to chill a little."

Chill out. If you don't have time to lollygag in the locker room, Dr. Dvorine suggests that you chill out—literally.

"It's okay to start with a warm shower, but you need to gradually reduce the amount of hot water until you're taking a cool shower," he says. "Cooler water will bring down your body temperature faster and reduce the likelihood of your sweating after you're dressed."

Skip a day. The quickest shower is none at all, and that's fine. "Some people feel that they must shower every day, or even several times a day," Dr. Levine says. "But it's not necessary. You can shower a few times a week and just wash your armpits and groin area each day to remove the bacteria. In fact, the more you shower, the more likely you'll dry out your skin, especially during the colder months."

Moisturize. Some guys would sooner ask for directions than apply moisturizer. But what may wound your machismo can help your skin, especially if you regularly shower after a workout.

"The key is to put on moisturizer immediately after your shower, while you're still wet," says Dr. Levine. "Moisturizing is good for everyone, but it's even more important if you shower frequently."

No Shower? No Sweat!

Don't sweat it if you don't have access to a shower after your midday workout.

"Those handy wipes that you get when you eat at a barbecue restaurant are a good way to remove sweat and clean yourself off," says Dr. William Dvorine, formerly of St. Agnes Hospital. "You can use them all over your body, and although they contain alcohol, it's no worse than the alcohol in antiperspirants. Since most of the offensive sweat is in your underarms and groin area, you can go to a bathroom and wash those areas, or any others, with these wipes."

Sorry, guys, but that's not a license to pig out on fatty ribs every week. The wipes also are sold in most supermarkets and other places that carry diapers and baby goods.

Carrying a small sponge in your workout bag is another good idea, adds Dr. Norman Levine of the University of Arizona College of Medicine. "Give yourself a sponge bath if you don't have a shower," he says. "You can easily do this in any sink."

Finally, there's the old cover-up. "Colognes, perfumes—there are a whole bunch of products that will mask the odor that results from sweating," Dr. Dvorine says. "Unless, you have a severe body odor problem, they are usually effective enough."

And for cleaning hair without a shower, No Water Needed is a nationally distributed "waterless" shampoo available at many drugstores and through mail-order. Just massage it into your hair, wait a few minutes, and comb out the dirt. It sells for about $6 for a 16-ounce bottle. For ordering and product information, call 1-800-248-8033.

Do-It-Yourself Exercise Equipment

Finding the Right Tools

You say that you'll let nothing come between you and your quest for perfect pecs. But there really are some things that make it impossible to get to the gym. Hurricanes, blizzards, medical quarantines, and house arrest come to mind.

Still, thanks to good old-fashioned human ingenuity, there's never a need to miss a workout. Because when you really think about it, the world itself is your gymnasium, and everything you see is a potential training tool.

You Might As Well Jump

You want to work out—you really do—but there's no exercise equipment in sight. At the end of your rope? Good. That's precisely where you should be. Now, go ahead and jump.

For a super aerobic workout that requires no expensive equipment and can be done in a confined space, jumping rope can't be beat. Ken Solis, M.D., author of *Ropics*, says basic rope jumping at 130 jumps per minute burns the same number of calories as running 9- to 10-minute miles.

"It's good to buy a real jump rope—most sporting-goods stores have them," says professional jump roper Louis Garcia of FreeStyle Roping, a company that promotes a new, "freestyle" form of jumping rope

that combines traditional jumping rope with dance and music, located in Burbank, California. "But in a pinch, you can make a jump rope out of almost any rope. It just has to be relatively thin, like a clothesline and have a slight amount of weight so that it keeps its shape and rotates easily."

Before you tear down the clothesline in the backyard, there are a few things that you should know. Like where you're going to dry your clothes now that you don't have a place to hang them outside. We can't help you with that one. But we can offer some advice on what to do with the rope.

First, make sure that it's customized for you. "Before you even start jumping, check the length," Garcia says. "Put one foot on the middle of the rope and pull up on it. Both ends should be chest-high—right about where your armpits are."

The same advice goes for buying a jump rope. Garcia recommends buying one adjustable in length.

Once the rope fits, you're ready to jump. Here's how, according to Garcia.

Stand on a mat or wooden floor with your feet together in front of the rope. Your hands should be just below your waist, your elbows close to your sides. The trick is to use only your wrists and forearms to swing the rope over your head and down in front of you. Try it. As the rope falls in front of you, jump one to two inches off the floor so that it can pass under. Land on the balls of your feet so that the impact is absorbed by your calves, rather than your shins and knees.

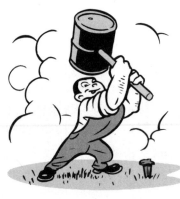

Start out trying to jump rope for about 2 minutes without missing. Slowly build up to 5, then 10, then 15 minutes.

Former world middleweight boxing contender Michael Olajidé, Jr., creator and author of *Aerobox: A High-Performance Fitness Program*, says,

"In just 15 minutes, you get a tremendous workout that will make your heart rate soar. It works your upper and lower body, and you barely have to leave the ground."

Once you've mastered the basic movement, try this twist suggested by Patrick Avon, founder of the Sergeant's Fitness Program near Washington, D.C.: Change your grip. Instead of holding the rope handles palms up, grab them palms down, thumbs facing in. This small adjustment takes the wrists out of the movement and forces you to use the muscles of your upper back and shoulders to spin the rope.

The great thing about jumping rope is that it can be done almost anytime, anywhere.

"Jump ropes are the ultimate portable workout," Garcia says. "You can pack a jump rope and take it with you anywhere."

Towel Off

Before you take down the clothesline, you might want to grab one of the towels off it. You'll be hard-pressed to find a more versatile piece of training equipment. Think about it. You can stretch with it, strengthen with it, and even wipe your brow when you're finished.

"It's possible to perform various isometric exercises by draping a towel around immovable things and pulling against them from different positions," says Alan Mikesky, Ph.D., an exercise physiologist and director of the Human Performance and Biochemistry Laboratory at Indiana University-Purdue University in Indianapolis. "But generally, towels work best in partner training, where you work with someone of comparable strength."

Here are some sample exercises suggested by Dr. Mikesky.

Performing under Pressure

If stress already has you clenching your fists all day, it's definitely time to get a grip—on reality.

"Relaxation exercises will make you realize that you don't have to adapt to the fast pace of the work environment," says Robert Delulio, Ed.D., a licensed counseling psychologist, certified personal trainer, and a licensed massage therapist in Madison, New Hampshire.

Assuming that your company doesn't have an onsite masseuse, you can settle for some self-administered acupressure. All you'll need to loosen up are a few tennis or racquetball balls, a sock, and a dowel.

When you're able to take a 10- to 15-minute break from your work, put two tennis or racquetball balls into the sock and tie the end, Dr. Delulio says. Then lie on your back with the balls behind the hollow spot on your upper neck, where they'll touch the ridge at the bottom of the skull.

"Once you hit the pressure points there, the musculature down the entire spine will begin to relax," Dr. Delulio says.

Alternatively, you can place the balls under any part of the back that is causing you discomfort, he says. "Anywhere you can feel pressure lying on them, you'll relieve stress in that area," he says.

Dr. Delulio suggests using this downtime to practice visualization. Just close your eyes and imagine yourself in a favorite place, concentrating on all five senses. Such relaxation exercises provide deep rest in small time periods, he says.

• Biceps curl: Hold the middle of the towel in one hand, with your arm straight out, palm up. Bend at the elbow to curl the arm upward while your partner kneels beside you and holds the ends of the towel and pulls downward to provide resistance.

• Seated row: Sit on the floor facing your partner, with the soles of your feet touching his. Begin with your arms outstretched, each of you using both hands to hold an opposite end of the towel. Then pull your arms toward your chest, squeezing your shoulder blades together, while your partner resists your pulling.

• Lower-back exercise: Begin in the same position as the seated row, but instead of bending your arms, lower your back toward the floor while your partner resists. Then your partner lowers his back and pulls you up as you resist.

• Hamstring curl: Stand with one hand resting on a desk for balance. Wrap the center of the towel around the back of your ankle. Bend at the knee to lift your heel toward your buttocks while your partner, who kneels beside you, holds the ends of the towel down toward the floor and provides resistance.

Dr. Mikesky warns that these exercises aren't easy to learn but says that they're useful for people who refuse to miss a workout—even when there aren't weights around.

"It takes practice to learn how to provide the other person proper resistance," Dr. Mikesky says. "You don't want him to have to stall out in the middle of a rep. Movements should be very smooth, never jerky. But it can be done, and it will be very effective."

Calling for the Squeeze Play

Once you have a towel in hand, you shouldn't miss those expensive gripper gizmos either. By simply rolling up some terry cloth and clenching it for a few seconds, you can strengthen your fingers and hands, says Steven Bogard, a physical therapist at the Mayo Clinic Hand Center in Rochester, Minnesota.

If you prefer, you could squeeze a soft sponge or a foam ball—or even just wad some sheets of paper and crunch them in your hand.

Whatever you use, Bogard suggests that you precede your grip work with some range-of-motion exercises. Curl your fingers, then spread them as far as you can. Stretch your wrist back and then down.

"This can help reduce hand cramps and get you limber," Bogard says.

If you do your hand workout regularly, not only will you improve your grip but you also might protect your hands from overuse syndrome.

"One of the main reasons these exercises are helpful is that they allow you to take a break from repetitive activities at your desk," Bogard says. "You just need to be careful not to make the exercises themselves repetitive. Anything you do to add variety to your hands' work has the capacity to enhance their ability to perform if you don't overwork them."

Getting a Lift

Strength building, in general, can be the perfect forum for creativity. After all, men have been known to bench-press everything from hotel end tables to their wives. (Not that we recommend either.)

Plenty of people reach for a book or paperweight and flex their arms while they're on the phone. While this probably wouldn't do much for Sylvester Stallone's physique, it can help older or beginning exercisers.

If you're a cost-conscious consumer, you might fill empty gallon milk jugs with varying levels of sand, as a substitute for a set of dumbbells—just be sure to keep caps on the containers, suggests Dr. Mikesky.

But no matter what you're using, it helps to know whether you're lifting the right amount.

"If your goal is to increase muscle strength, you want to lift a load that you can only perform 10 to 15 repetitions with while maintaining good form," Dr. Mikesky says.

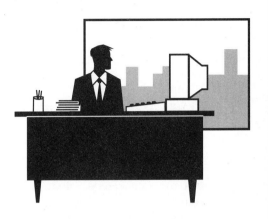

Part Five

Real-Life Scenarios

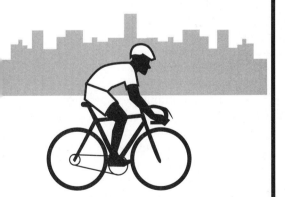

Quest for the Best

They're successful, celebrated, and at the top of their games. And they share one other thing in common: Each of these men carves time out of his jam-packed schedule to work out regularly.

You Can Do It!

They work hard, just like you. They also work out hard to stay in top shape. So can you.

Male Makeovers

Finding the time for exercise—and getting the most out of it when you do—isn't easy. So we turned to the experts for their best advice for some common scenarios. See if any sound familiar.

Quest for the Best They're successful, celebrated, and at the top of their games. And they share one other thing in common: Each of these men carves time out of his jam-packed schedule to work out regularly.

Pat O'Brien, CBS Sportscaster

From Tragedy to Triumph

A lot of things changed for Pat O'Brien the day his best friend died of a heart attack at age 48. Not the least of which was his commitment to fitness.

"It's a wake-up call," says O'Brien, who is in his late forties. "I think that, deep inside, all men fear getting through that middle-age part of life—between ages 47 and 52. Out of the corner of your eye you start reading those obits—and you see guys with two kids falling over with heart attacks. That sticks with you. And if something unfortunate happens close to you, it hits even harder."

Stung by the tragedy, the gregarious sportscaster decided to examine his own health habits. "I always thought that I was in pretty good shape. But frankly, I wasn't. I was thin and all that, but I wasn't lean. I'd run a little bit here and there, and that was it."

If anyone could muster a credible excuse not to exercise, it would be a guy like O'Brien. Lead CBS broadcaster for such grueling events as the National Collegiate Athletic Association (NCAA) Basketball Tournament and the Winter Olympics, host of both a daily sports radio show, a weekly online sports report, and guest host of Entertainment Tonight—not to mention a travel schedule that rivals a U.N. peacekeeper (he lives in Los Angeles with his wife, Linda, and son, Sean)—no one

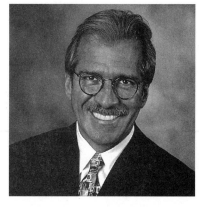

would blame O'Brien if he simply hung a "No Housekeeping" sign on his hotel door and snoozed until his next on-air appearance.

A Man with a Workout Plan

Enter personal trainer Pete Steinfeld. Soon after his friend's death, O'Brien undertook an exercise program that rivals nearly any in its focus on intensity and abdominal strengthening.

"The workout I do with Pete is a killer. He watches my form and readies equipment so that I can go from one exercise to the next without stopping. It works all my muscles. As a result, I'm in the best shape of my life—six-foot-one, 167 pounds with about 8 percent body fat."

But before O'Brien even thinks about touching a weight, he hits the road for a three- to five-mile morning run—even when he's traveling. "I get it out of the way early so that if I do get backed up, I won't have to skip a workout," he says. "The run also helps me see different parts of cities that I am working in—places where I normally wouldn't go."

Back at the hotel or his home, O'Brien warms up with a series of movements designed to increase circulation, including neck rolls, extended arm circles, trunk twists, broomstick twists (broomstick on the shoulder, torso twist), and side bends.

Next it's on to abdominal exercises, including side bends and bicycle, bent-knee, and straight-leg crunches. O'Brien can now knock off 1,000 total reps in about 9 or 10 minutes.

Then, in an effort to maintain muscle balance and symmetry, O'Brien works his upper body and arms, doing high-rep sets of push-ups, dumbbell bench presses, barbell bent-over rows, seated dumbbell military presses, seated alternating dumbbell curls, seated triceps dumbbell extensions, and ankle squats. Sometimes he splits the routine so that he's only doing half the weight exercises. The total workout time, on a good day, is about 36 minutes.

When in Los Angeles, O'Brien also visits a fitness class called Tae Bo aerobics, run by martial arts expert and actor Billy Blanks. A mixture of kickboxing, boxing, and aerobics, O'Brien joined after some ribbing from his pals: former boxing champion Sugar Ray Leonard and hockey great Wayne Gretzky.

"They said, 'You think you're in shape? C'mon over here,' " says O'Brien. "For a full hour you're throwing punches and kicks, moving all the time, bouncing up and down. You work so hard that your eyelids sweat. If you can do this, you're in shape, period, exclamation point."

Most men claim that they work out harder when they have a training partner. With athletes the caliber of Leonard, Gretzky, and former Olympic decathlon gold medalist Bruce Jenner in class, O'Brien has even more motivation.

"I prefer to run alone, but I like to be in the gym with these guys interacting and getting it done," says O'Brien.

The Tournament Test

A Sioux Falls, South Dakota, native, O'Brien began his broadcasting career in 1970 after he graduated from the University of South Dakota. His first job was as a researcher at NBC News in Washington, D.C. He later worked as a reporter at WMAQ-TV in Chicago and in 1977 moved to the CBS affiliate in Los Angeles.

After earning four local Emmy Awards for news coverage, O'Brien made the jump to the network sports team in 1981. During his

CBS career, O'Brien has covered many of the most prestigious sporting events in the world, including the Super Bowl, the NBA Finals, the World Series, the U.S. Open Tennis Championships, and the World Figure Skating Championships.

Few events, however, test O'Brien's commitment to fitness like the NCAA Basketball Tournament, affectionately known as March Madness. On a typical day during the tournament, O'Brien arrives at about 10:00 A.M. and works until midnight.

"No matter how late I'm up, I always wake up in the morning between 5:30 A.M. and 6:00 A.M., flip on *Imus in the Morning* (the controversial syndicated radio show), and run from 57th Street in New York City to 95th Street and back. Or run through Central Park to Harlem and back."

Instead of heading straight for his room after his run, O'Brien hits the hotel gym. "That's where I do a little stretching, ab work, and strengthening," he says. "If you're in your room and you've done 10 push-ups and sit-ups and the phone rings and you are on the phone for 15 minutes, you've blown your workout."

Between calling games and tapings, O'Brien says that he'll nurse a Coke and sometimes chat with the crew about training techniques. And he speaks with half-serious pride about a movement to get the network to add salad to the standard meal of pizza and other goodies they provide.

"Pizza tastes pretty good when you have been on the air all day. You can eat a lot if you're not careful," he says. "If anyone tells you that they eat well on the road, they're lying to you. If I have to eat something completely unhealthy, I'll eat only half of it."

It's that kind of commitment to fitness that O'Brien believes is the key to staying in shape.

"You never find time. You make time. I really believe that it's a force of habit. You have to get into something so much that once you start doing it and stop, you'll almost feel guilty."

Thomas R. Carper, Governor of Delaware

A Lifetime Commitment to Fitness

Delaware is so small, you can drive from one tip to the other in a little more than two hours. When you do, you'll pass through all three of the state's counties. It has just one representative in Congress and only one area code.

Dwarfed by the surrounding states of Pennsylvania, New Jersey, and Maryland, Delaware for years pitched itself to tourists as Small Wonder. Now, in these more competitive times, it bills itself as the home of tax-free shopping, hoping that its lack of a sales tax will lure shoppers across state lines, an approach that seems to be working. Perhaps Delaware would call more attention to itself if it were the smallest state in the nation. But with just slightly more than 1,900 square miles, it's larger than Rhode Island. And with 706,000 people, it's more populated than Alaska and several other states.

Delaware's diminutive size, however, does not make it any less challenging to govern. Just ask Gov. Thomas R. Carper, who puts an average of 14 hours a day into keeping fresh ink on the law books, police cars on the roads, sand on the coastline, pollution out of the inland bays, banks and other big companies within the state boundaries, and traffic from clogging up the small towns that have the misfortune of being located along beach routes jammed by summer tourists.

Splitting his time between his home in Wilmington and the Governor's mansion in the state capital of Dover, Carper's life outside of work is just as demanding as his job. He's the devoted father of two young boys. Still, hardly a day goes by that he doesn't squeeze a workout into his hectic workday.

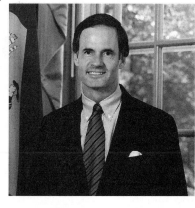

Hitting the Gym

On a perfect day, Carper gets up by 6:00 A.M. and works for an hour or so. Then he gets his sons, Christopher and Ben, out of bed, makes them breakfast, and sends them to school. Finally, he heads over to the YMCA for a workout.

"It gives me energy," says Carper, who has maintained his boyish good looks into his late forties. "It puts me in a great mood for the rest of the day. All kinds of things can go wrong. Sometimes everything goes wrong. But after a morning workout, I will still have a good day."

Like most of us, though, Carper doesn't enjoy many perfect days. Often he has an early meeting to run off to. In that case he'll fit in his workout whenever there's an open space in his schedule. When in Wilmington, he alternates between two YMCAs. When in Dover, he opts for the Dover Air Force Base gym or the Dover YMCA. All four gyms offer flexible hours, with the Air Force Base the most accommodating. "I hate gyms that have lousy hours," says Carper, a retired naval fight officer. "There was a time that the Dover Air Force Base gym opened at 5:00 A.M. and closed at 2:00 A.M.," he says. Now that's customer service.

Flexible gym hours are important for a busy governor who has worked out as late as 11:00 P.M. Carper usually works out every day. On Monday through Saturday, he rotates twice through a three-day routine that includes weight lifting, stair-stepping, and stationary cycling. When on the stair-climber or stationary bike, Carper tries to burn 500 calories, which usually takes a half-hour to 45 minutes. Weight lifting usually takes 45 minutes.

On Sundays, Carper either runs about 6 miles in Wilmington at an eight-minute-mile pace or bikes 20 miles through the Amish farm country if he's staying in Dover. Either way, he's out on the road by 7:00 A.M. and home in time to make his wife, Martha, and sons breakfast before heading for church.

"I used to run every other day," Carper says. "But I've talked to people who run a lot, and eventually their knees and ankles give out on them. So I've decided to do things that are probably not as tough on my legs but still get the heart pumping and the blood circulating."

Though he only runs one day a week, Carper still makes sure that he gets in shape each year for the Caesar Rodney Half-Marathon, a 13.1 mile race held every March over a challenging, hilly course in Wilmington. Instead of running more often, he just runs longer on Sundays. "Starting in January, I'll add a mile a week. Instead of running 6 miles, one week I'll run 7, the next 8. I'll stretch it out so by the time the Caesar Rodney rolls around, I can run 13 miles without too much pain," says Carper.

On the Move

Even when he's on the road, Carper makes time for exercise. Sometimes that means that his staff must sweat it out with him.

During one West Coast trip, Carper and his staff arrived at the San Francisco airport at noon, drove into San Francisco, parked under the Bank of America building (where he would later have a meeting), walked three blocks to the Chinatown YMCA, worked out, showered, and then walked back to the bank for the 2:00 P.M. meeting.

That night, Carper flew to Portland, Oregon. He got up at 6:30 A.M. and worked out at an athletic club two blocks from the hotel, then went to a meeting. "I always find a place to go work out," says Carper. "Sometimes the hotels have facilities. Other times I have to scout around. If there's no place open, I'll just run."

Staying Shipshape

Carper has kept himself in good shape since his early Navy days. At age 21 he graduated from Ohio State University and became an ensign in the Navy at Pensacola, Florida. Though he was in pretty good shape all through college, the Navy put him in the best shape of his life. During preflight training, Carper did countless calisthenics, obstacle courses, and running.

"I got to be in real good shape. And I liked the way it felt," Carper says. "I sort of made a promise to myself that for as long as I could, I wanted to stay in that kind of shape. And for the most part I have."

Even when he wasn't forced to exercise, Carper made sure to work out at various military gyms during his Naval career. He ran the roads and backstreets of countries all over the world. And when he left the Navy in 1973 to attend graduate school at the University of Delaware, Carper made sure to visit the university gym early and often.

The Democrat has managed to keep up the routine through a successful political career that has seen him rise from state treasurer to congressman to governor.

Exercise helps Carper relieve stress, stay healthy, and look younger and better. It energizes him. And it helps him become the father he strives to be.

"We had our kids later in life," Carper says. "I like being able to do things with them—sports, athletics. One of the benefits of me staying in shape is that we can play soccer, basketball, and baseball. I can just have a great time with my kids."

Because exercise improves his life so much, Carper has rarely had a day where he has had trouble motivating himself.

"I have just made this a part of my life for over 20 years," Carper says. "If I miss it more than a day, I feel guilty and I feel lousy. A combination of those two feelings will get me back on track quickly."

David Bradley, Author

Writing on the Run

David Bradley's life is jammed.

The acclaimed author sometimes works on more than one book at a time while he free-lances for newspapers and magazines, lectures at various colleges and writers' organizations around the country, and even works on a movie deal. He splits his time between two homes: one in Philadelphia, another in La Jolla, California. He spends many nights in hotels and is often on the road or in the air.

But he manages to find time to run—for at least an hour on most days. And he lifts weights a couple days a week. For Bradley, skipping workouts because he's too busy is not an option. Now in his mid-forties, Bradley has been running for more than 25 years.

"The only serious time I have been down is when I was injured," says the author of *South Street* and *The Chaneysville Incident*, which won the 1982 PEN/Faulkner Award. In 1980, Bradley blew out a knee after competing in nu-merous marathons. The injury did take away some of his competitiveness. But it didn't stop him from running.

"The idea that I might not ever run again is just not there. Even when I have been sick and not able to run for a couple weeks, there's always the question of how soon I can get back to it. I think that's just something that comes with a lot of years of doing it and realizing that it's part of my life," says Bradley.

The Big Decision

Hard as it is to imagine, Bradley's life is actually less hectic than it once was. In the mid-1970s he worked as an ed-itor at J. B. Lippincott in New York City, spending about 70

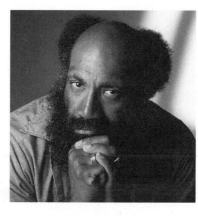

hours a week at the office. He was under tremendous stress, but he managed to go to a track over by the East River and run three days a week. Sometimes, if he was lucky, he could fit it in after work. But he couldn't run too late in the evening. "In New York, you don't want to be going over there at 7:00 or 8:00 at night," Bradley says.

Time flew by, and so did the miles. Looking back, he can't figure out exactly how he fit it all in. But eventually, the frenzied pace caught up with him. His running had become stressful. He felt pressured to run faster so that he could get other things done.

Faced with a choice between running and work, Bradley decided to quit his job.

"I had been editing a book on running (*The Joy of Running*). The author (Thaddeus Kostrubala) was writing about running marathons. I decided that I wanted to do that. Something had to go. So the job gave," says Bradley.

Creative Running

Though his new life of freelance writing and lecturing allowed Bradley to pretty much set his own schedule, it didn't give him tons of free time. Just traveling to various speaking en-gagements involves sitting in airports, on airplanes, and in cars—all time that could be spent running. And writing novels isn't exactly a speedy process.

So it's a good thing that Bradley can work while he runs.

"What I do for a living, of course, has a lot to do with thinking. You can think anywhere. You don't have to be doing anything with your hands while you are thinking. In fact, I think it is more beneficial to be away from the word processor while you are trying to work through various problems. As those things come up in your mind, you work through them without having to commit to the paper or the word processor," says Bradley.

Often, Bradley sits at his keyboard and types. Then, silence. Maybe it's a plot that has run out of options. Or a character who needs to say something but has contracted verbal amnesia. Or maybe it's a speech that needs a third main point. The silence all means the same thing—it's time to run.

It takes about 20 to 30 minutes before the answers start coming, before the characters start talking, the plots start turning around, and the outlines start changing.

"In your mind you have an outline somewhere. You get committed to that. You are sitting there trying desperately to work it out," Bradley says. "Then you get away from it. You go out and run for 15 to 20 minutes, and suddenly it hits you that you don't have to do it that way at all. Things that you have not thought of, things that are hard to think of while you are in the middle of something, come to you."

Bradley is not sure why the running technique works. Maybe it's because it makes him so relaxed. Or maybe it's the endorphin rush. Or maybe it's the fact that when he's on the run, no idea is a bad idea.

"It's just the inability to act on something. In society we tend to act on our ideas immediately. We're under a lot of pressure to do that. And running is a context where you can't act immediately. You are five miles out. Before you can do anything, you have to come five miles back. It just forces you to go through things or to rehearse things," Bradley says.

The same thing can't be said for weight lifting. Bradley doesn't think up characters, plots, or outlines while he pumps iron. But working out with weights has helped him save time on the job. "The weights are good for meetings. If I know that it is going to be a tense or difficult situation, I will work out ahead of time. That way, I blow off a lot of the tension that I anticipate," he says.

After lifting weights, Bradley can walk into a meeting calm, prepared to present his side in a nonthreatening manner. And all concerned can discuss options and come to a consensus rather than increasing the tension to such a level that everyone begins hurling invective.

"People ask me if I work out because I want to live forever. I tell them that I work out because I want them to live forever," Bradley says.

Making Time

Even though both aspects of his exercise routine help him do his job, Bradley still struggles to fit them in. When on the road, he sometimes splits weight lifting into multiple workouts. For instance, during a spare 15 minutes he'll do push-ups. During another break he'll do crunches.

Over the years, Bradley has gotten pretty creative at turning a hotel room into a miniature gym. He uses chairs to do decline push-ups. And he uses chairs and other furniture as his weights.

"It's kind of hard to come up with something that is the equivalent of a 220-pound bench press. But it can be done. I do military presses with chairs. I hold the chair over my head. If a maid happens to come in at that moment, things can get a little weird," Bradley says with a laugh.

But Bradley can't break up his running routine. If he doesn't have enough time to run, he will walk instead.

"It doesn't do me any good to run for less than an hour. It just doesn't. It isn't worth it," Bradley says. "I'm trained to run a distance of 10 to 12 miles. Three miles just gets me going. It's not really a lot of fun for me to run under pressure. I like to do it away from pressure. So when I'm really pressured and I don't have the time to do it right, I'll put running off. But there's a limit. Sooner or later I'll say, 'Sorry guys, I gotta go.' "

Gary Barnett, Northwestern University Football Coach

Running for the Roses

Being a miracle worker has a way of keeping a guy busy.

Just look at Gary Barnett, the man who turned the once hopelessly pathetic Northwestern University football team into a Big 10 conference champion.

How'd he do it? By working 15 hours a day, seven days a week; by telling anyone and everyone that his team was going to succeed—no matter how often people laughed in his face; by staking a claim on a program that everyone else had given up on.

"We were in the epitome of a situation where you want to feel like you can't change the system," he says. "But what we did is *prove* that no matter where you are, you are in control. Most of us prefer to point fingers somewhere else and say, 'That's the reason I'm not where I want to be.' But you really do have control. You have to believe that, because if you choose to look at it the other way, you'll be right. You'll never make a difference."

Exercising Control

Barnett's "no excuses" philosophy extends directly to his personal fitness regime. While some of his head-coaching counterparts look as though they're living on double cheeseburgers and cigars, Barnett, now in his early fifties, has made his health a high priority.

It all started when he took up running in 1976, and it gained momentum when he drastically reduced his red meat consumption two years later.

"During the season, now, I really watch my diet—especially during two-a-days," he says. "In the morning I have fruit. At noon I have salad. And in the evening I make sure that I get my vegetables. I try not to eat anything after dinner."

When it comes to strength training, Barnett prefers to do things the old-fashioned way: alternating each morning between doing 60 push-ups or 200 sit-ups. He keeps his aerobic exercise simple, too, especially when he has to make recruiting trips in December and January.

"I don't really like the other exercise machines, but I do try to stay at places that have treadmills," he says. "Otherwise what I can do depends on where I have to go. If I go south or west, I can usually run outside. But if I'm in the Northeast or the Midwest that time of year, it's very hard."

The weather may not always cooperate with his plans, but at least Barnett's body is holding up. While a lot of men his age are hobbled by old football injuries, Barnett managed to emerge relatively unscathed from his playing days at the University of Missouri in the late 1960s. Though he's had knee surgery and sometimes contends with a troublesome calf muscle, he has no chronic aches or pains that would interfere with his workouts.

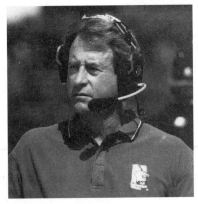

That means that almost nothing can keep him from a 3½-mile run, six days a week.

"It's aerobic obviously, but honestly, I do it for my head," he says. "It gets me a break in the middle of the day. I walk out the door with all my problems, and by the time I'm finished, they're solved. I just try to get into an unconscious state. I usually do not even know where I have run."

Running Out the Clock

Barnett cherishes the chance to clear his head, because the rest of his day is a study in time micromanagement. From the beginning of August to Thanksgiving, there are no days off—just a never-ending stream of decisions to make and questions to answer.

Practice days begin with a 7:00 A.M. meeting of the full coaching staff, to coordinate plans and discuss personnel issues. From 8:00 A.M. to 11:00 A.M., Barnett sits in on strategy sessions with either the offensive or defensive staffs.

"At these meetings, our goal is to make a plan for each potential game situation—for instance, what we are going to do this week on second and long," he says. "We make these decisions based on the game films and what we see at practice."

Fans who think that this process sounds more like fun than work are mistaken.

"You would be amazed at the amount of time that goes into just planning a practice," Barnett says. "We watch video on each opponent that's broken down by computers to chart their tendencies. And we do the same thing to ourselves, to be aware of what other people are looking at as our own tendencies."

One off-field tendency that Barnett is known for is his prompt, direct dealings with members of the media. He leaves a two-hour block open for interviews, beginning at 11:00 A.M. By 1:00 P.M. he's ready to run.

When he returns from his workout at 2:00 P.M., the coaches meet for a final review of the afternoon's practice schedule, which begins with a brief team meeting at 2:45 P.M. From there, players break off into position meetings. Everyone takes the field at 3:40 P.M.

"We script every minute of practice," Barnett says. "In every 10-minute interval, we run 15 plays. Every one of those plays has a purpose. It's been thought through carefully. We can't afford to fall behind."

Things are scheduled to wrap up at 6:00 P.M. Barnett often takes questions from reporters and fans who attend practice, then eats dinner with the team. His work isn't done, though.

"At 7:00 P.M., I come back to my office and make recruiting calls or put on the practice film from that afternoon," he says. "I generally finish up after 9:30 P.M. and get home at about 10:00 P.M."

All in the Family

The in-season schedule obviously doesn't allow for much time at home with his wife, Mary. Off-seasons are somewhat more relaxed, though there are still clinics and camps to run—and award ceremonies to attend. But Barnett says that his children—son, Clay, and daughter, Courtney, now both in college—have benefited from his career in football, although he acknowledges that his family life may not be what most people would consider normal.

"I don't know if someone on the outside can understand it, but college football is a way of life for a coach's family," he says. "Everything revolves around football. Instead of taking family vacations, you go to bowl games."

Well, they do now. But during Barnett's first three seasons at Northwestern—in which his teams won a total of eight games—the Wildcats didn't look to be any closer to a bowl bid than they'd been in any other year since their 1949 Rose Bowl victory. That didn't sit well with Barnett, who believed that he was building a better program, not just adding to the school's losing tradition.

"That pressure is very personal," he says. "It's the pride of wanting to do a good job, knowing that every Saturday your work is laid out in front of everybody. People do judge you based on your wins and losses."

For Barnett, coping with success is a lot more fun.

"When you go 24 years without a winning season, *that's* pressure," he says. "There may be more expectations for us now, but I do not equate expectations to pressure."

Doug Colbeth, Spyglass Chief Executive Officer

On the Go with the Web Runner

One year Doug Colbeth didn't know if he could make his house payments. The next year he had a net worth in the tens of millions of dollars.

The Spyglass president and chief executive officer is one of many small-business men who've cashed in on the current computer craze. But sudden success has also meant megastress, and Colbeth has found that making time for fitness is essential for keeping his life on track.

Though probably best known for its commercial version of the University of Illinois World Wide Web browser Mosaic, Spyglass provides a suite of embedded networking technologies for the products of more than 100 companies, including Microsoft and IBM.

"Our goal is to be inside with 2,000 products by the year 2000," Colbeth says. "We want to get World Wide Web technologies into the hands of all the people in the world who do *not* use computers."

Spyglass, headquartered in Naperville, Illinois, has offices in four U.S. cities and is expanding into Europe and Asia. Since the company's breakthrough in 1994, the number of employees has been doubling every year, while profits have continued to soar.

All that has meant a worldwide web of responsibility for Colbeth, who works as many as 15 hours a day and spends much of his life in airports and hotel rooms.

"My personal life has suffered some," says Colbeth, now in his early forties. "Not with my kids, because I would never sacrifice that. But I have sacrificed what I would call pure fun. My golf is terrible, and

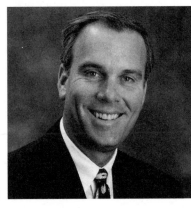

I miss it. But I believe that I'm making a temporary trade-off."

A Running Start

Colbeth may have lost his grip on his golf clubs, but he firmly grasps the importance of a healthy lifestyle. His average day begins with a 5:30 A.M. jog.

On weekdays, Colbeth puts in 4 to 5 miles on the treadmill or the track. "I plan my workouts a week ahead, based on what my schedule looks like," he says. "I'm looking to get in 20 miles a week over four to five days. I may miss a day if I'm taking an early-morning flight, but then I always run the next day."

Colbeth says that he feels lethargic on days when he misses his morning run.

"I feel more alert after I jog, and that feeling lasts all day," he says. "Obviously, it's most intense right after a workout, but I feel good even toward the latter part of the day. Everyone has optimistic and pessimistic sides, and my optimistic side comes out much more with regular exercise."

That's why the Colbeths keep a treadmill, a stair-climber, and weights in the room over their garage—in what was once Spyglass headquarters.

"Time is very important. I don't even go to health clubs anymore because of the 15 minutes you spend going each way. But I can always roll out of bed and get on a treadmill."

A former football player, the six-foot-two, 210-pound executive still lifts weights three times a week to tone his arms, doing high repetitions with relatively light weights. But he considers running to be the mainstay of his fitness routine.

"Jogging works for me because I'm not depending on someone else," he says. "True, a racquetball game would be more fun, and I love to play basketball in the driveway with my son. But that's not something you can do when you travel. Those are just fun weekend things."

Colbeth follows his morning run with a breakfast packed with plenty of fiber and fruit. By 7:30 A.M. he's on his way to the office or the airport. Either way, he can look forward to a day of constant discussion with customers, potential partners, and fellow executives.

"I often have speaking engagements, which are typically around noon," Colbeth says. "I don't like to eat before I speak, and usually, the meal is cold by the time I'm done talking, so I don't end up eating much."

To compensate, he'll reach for some fruit between his afternoon meetings, which are scheduled in precise 30-minute blocks. Work tends to extend into the evening, especially during the two or three days a week he typically spends on the road.

"Over the years, I've learned that I need a very controlled diet when I travel or else it's much more exhausting," he says. "At first, I ate too much and drank too much. Now I'm much more careful. I don't drink alcohol on the road, and I don't eat late-night meals. I eat at 6:00 P.M. or 7:00 P.M., then schedule a meeting after dinner. That way I don't go to bed on a full stomach."

With his stomach settled, Colbeth can turn to settling his mind. He insists on having an hour to himself before getting his 6½ hours of sleep.

"The two sane hours of my life are when I'm running in the morning and at 10:00 P.M.," he says. "I'm a sports fanatic, so I catch the nightly wrap-up on ESPN. But I'm always in bed by 11:00 P.M., because if I try to function on three to four hours of sleep, I really start dragging at the end of the next day.

Working Things Out

Organizing a training schedule is a tiny challenge compared to some that Colbeth has faced. As recently as 1994, Spyglass was on the verge of going broke, and his family didn't know how—or if—they'd be able to pay the three

mortgages they had taken out on their house.

"I used to wake up in cold sweats a lot of nights," he says. "There were three things that were really gnawing at me. One was that we'd gone through the savings for our kids' college. Second was that I felt like the employees were going to be let down if the company couldn't continue. Then there was the personal pressure of wanting to be successful."

Unable to find any solutions himself but unwilling to give up, he put his 17 employees in a room and asked them to brainstorm new markets and investors that Spyglass could pursue. From that meeting came the idea that would eventually earn the company millions.

"When you don't have anything, you really learn how to build partnerships," Colbeth says. "We had to build, first, with the employees. We had to let them be a part of deciding what to do next. Then we had to build with the University of Illinois. We told them: 'We have a great idea. You have a great technology with Mosaic. Let us take it over commercially.' "

Colbeth's relationships, at work and at home, remain the key to minimizing the pressure he feels as he tries to direct the company's frenzied growth.

"As my executive staff gets better, that takes stress off me," he says. "Two years ago I didn't have that infrastructure. Now I have the support staff that makes my days easier—not easy, but easier."

He's also learned that a social calendar can be as much of a strain as a business calendar. Colbeth and his wife, Margey, have two children—a daughter, Jackie, and son, Brett—who help keep them plenty busy.

But no matter what parts of his personal schedule are shuffled, one thing that Colbeth will never give up is his exercise.

"I want to contribute to this industry when I'm in my fifties and potentially in my sixties," he says. "To do that, I have to stay in shape in my forties. I look at those 45 minutes a day I run as an investment, so I'll have a longer career and feel better."

Tom Peters, Management Expert and Author

A Passion for Walking

Another exhausting five-day management seminar behind him, Tom Peters eased his 5-foot-11, 220-pound frame into a hotel chair and began reading comment cards from the participants—standard procedure after each event.

Among them was a two-sentence note from the chief financial officer of a huge health care organization. "Tom is a walking heart attack," it said. "Will give him a free stress test anytime he wants one."

The message cut through the management expert like a pink slip on Friday at 5:00 P.M. Peters knew that he was overweight and that his face turned beet red when he got worked up during a seminar. Heck, he'd even spit sometimes while talking to high-powered executives. And worst of all, he never could quite find time to exercise.

The next morning, Peters got up and took a nice, long walk—and liked it. Two days later he bought and read *Aerobic Walking* by Casey Meyers. "Life is weird. Why after X number of years of being a very irregular exerciser that particular line hit me, I have no idea. But with the exception of taking a 30-day hiatus a couple of times, I haven't stopped walking since," he says.

Trading Fitness for Success

It's not as if Peters had been standing still. His first book, *In Search of Excellence*, has sold more than five million

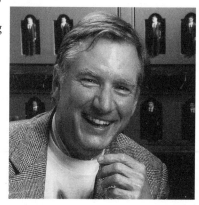

copies, and he also authored the bestsellers *A Passion for Excellence*, *Thriving on Chaos*, and *Liberation Management*. One of the nation's foremost authorities on business management, Peters wrote a syndicated newspaper column, penned the foreword to more than 30 books, authored articles for publications from *Business Week* and *The Economist* to the *Wall Street Journal* and *Harvard Business Review*, and founded the Tom Peters Group, three training and communications companies headquartered in Palo Alto, California.

But as we all know, busy doesn't mean fit. And when it came to physical activity, an occasional racquetball game was all the exercise this management expert could swing. And even then it wasn't managed very well. "Nothing about it was planned—it was a function of when a buddy had some free time," he says.

Peters's extensive travel schedule didn't help. With 150 to 160 management seminars a year—and stops in such far-flung locales as Düsseldorf, Paris, and Bangkok—keeping in shape was that much more difficult. Peters doesn't like jogging ("God bless the people who do," he says); hotel gyms aren't for him either. The bottom line is that, aside from the considerable energy he expended during the seminar, he wouldn't do much of anything.

And, although he rarely found himself overeating at mealtime, mini-bars seemed to get the best of him—particularly on Monday nights. "Lord help me during Monday Night Football," says Peters. "It's hard to stay away from the cashews. If memory serves, cashews are about 1,000 calories a bite, and you get your first 1,000-calorie hit when you just take the top off the bottle."

On the Right Path

But speed walking—or dork walking, as one of Peters's

friends likes to call it—was a perfect marriage of his busy schedule and his disdain for more formal exercise.

An early riser, Peters often decides when to walk based on the "terror quotient" of the city he's visiting. "I don't like walking in some cities when it's pitch dark and the middle of December," he says. "So I usually wait until dawn, or sometime between. It's a great way to start the day when I'm going to be in an intense seminar. I discovered that if I didn't do it at the crack of dawn, the statistical odds of me doing it went way down."

When he's at home—be it Palo Alto, California, or Tinmouth, Vermont (site of his 1,300-acre working farm)—Peters prefers an afternoon jaunt. "It probably doesn't happen more than 20 percent of the time, but I'll work until 1:00 P.M. and then take an hour walk to decompress," he says.

Just how long Peters walks also varies. Staying in cities like Cincinnati or Chicago only seems to allow 25-minute treks; a walk at home could last 90 minutes. "If it's a rotten, snowy day in Chicago and the wind is roaring off the lake and the temperature is -7°F, I'll go out for 10 minutes, and 10 minutes is just fine. It's the act of doing it and the consistency that's important," he says. "There's a feeling of arrogant, egocentric self-satisfaction about having beaten your way through a blizzard. The crappier the weather, the more I like it."

And the walk itself? Definitely "not a thing of beauty," he says. "I think that I have reasonably good arm form and body posture, but speed walking doesn't look too good unless it's being performed somewhere like the Olympics."

Unlike the Olympics, you'll never see Peters in a pack of other speed walkers. "If I ran into my best friend on earth in the lobby of the hotel and he said, 'Do you want to walk together?' I'll certainly walk around town with him, but I won't speed walk with him. That's my private thing that has nothing to do with any of my 6.2 billion fellow human beings."

Walking for Inspiration and Perspiration

In addition to all the physiological benefits of speed walking—Peters says that he's read that it works more muscles, burns more calories, and is easier on the joints than jogging—it has also become a source of inspiration for him.

"When I wrote my column, I would guess that roughly 40 percent of them were written on my walks—especially when I was totally out of ideas," he says. "Forty-eight hours before the damn thing was due, I would say that it's this walk or else. You walk until you get an idea. That didn't always work, but it worked reasonably well."

On topics relating to business and management, Peters is unabashedly outspoken. A biography provided by Peters describes him as a "gadfly, curmudgeon, champion of bold failures, prince of disorder, maestro of zest, professional loudmouth, corporate cheerleader, lover of markets, (and) capitalist pig." But he rarely chooses to share his enthusiasm for walking with others.

"I remember disliking being beaten up by the you-have-to-exercise people," Peters says. "If someone asks me about it, I'll tell them. But my shtick is business and business management."

Still, Peters credits walking with energizing his life and making him happier as well as healthier. "Walking really makes a physiological, chemical difference," he says. "If you crawled around the block, it would still be incredibly valuable. There's nothing more fun. It's rung just about every bell that you can find in my church spire."

Not only that, but he's 25 pounds lighter and has passed the last three stress tests without a hitch.

"A few years ago I tried to find that guy to thank him, and I never did. But I did take him up on his offer," says Peters. "Just not on the freebie."

You Can Do It! They work hard, just like you. They also work out hard to stay in top shape. So can you.

On the Run, On the Job

Richard Bishop, Winston, Georgia

Date of birth: May 30, 1959

Height and weight: 5-foot-11, 165 pounds

Profession: Welding and equipment repair

If someone told me a few years ago that I would run in the 100th anniversary of the Boston Marathon, I would have told them that they were flat out crazy. For most of my life, I wouldn't even run to the mailbox, if you know what I mean.

I guess I was what you'd call a couch potato. At 5-foot-11, I weighed about 200 pounds. And after working second shift maintenance at the General Motors (GM) plant in Atlanta—from 3:30 P.M. to midnight—about all I would do was go to bed. You can't do much when you get home except go to bed. Then I'd wake up around 9:00 A.M. or 10:00 A.M., eat breakfast, watch a little TV, do some chores around the house, eat lunch, and get ready for work. I have three kids—the oldest boy is 17, my middle boy is 15, and my little girl is 11—and I hardly ever saw them. They were in school by the time I woke up.

When I worked day shift, I'd come home, watch TV and eat supper, and whatever, but even then I wasn't very active.

I always tried to eat pretty healthy, but I have my weaknesses. I still like cookies and ice cream and stuff. But before I started running, I'd get going and eat way too much—any flavor of ice cream, it didn't matter. And I used to drink a lot of Coca-Cola and eat chips from out of the machine at work.

When I was a kid, we lived on a lake, and I water-skied and swam some. So I'd lose a little weight during the summer and then gain it

back in the winter. But I never ran in high school and, aside from little league baseball, never really played sports. I hadn't done any real exercise for years.

The First Step

Then one day I saw all this literature around the plant announcing a new health program called Live for Life. It said that a fitness center was opening and would offer programs to all the employees. I started thinking: I'm getting a little bit older. Maybe I need to take better care of myself.

Finally, I decided to go up there and try it out. Well, I started walking on the outside around the GM plant. And after a while, I'd jog a little bit and walk a little bit. You know, alternate. I set a goal to lose 20 pounds—a number that seemed about right for me.

Then I thought: Maybe if I got to work early I could go up there and work out and then come back up during my 30-minute break or at lunch. Well, I started getting up earlier and getting my workout in. By the end of the 12-week program, I had lost about 26 pounds. What convinced me to stick with it? I noticed that I had more energy and generally felt a lot better. I just got into it.

At about that time I saw a flyer for a 10-K race—the Heart Track '92 race in Atlanta. And I said well, let me try that out. I ran it in 42 minutes and something—a pretty fair showing for a first race.

Since then, I've been hooked. I ran about 25 races that year—5-Ks, 10-Ks, it didn't matter. And in about four years, I've run in more than 200 races, including four marathons and three half-marathons! I'm not sure why I like it so much. Maybe it's the thrill of competing. In fact, I haven't missed a day running in 13 to 14 months.

Making Time to Train

Of course, it's not exactly easy to train with my schedule. I'm on a 12-hour day shift now starting at 6:00 A.M. We have a break around 8:30 A.M., so I usually get out and run down the side of the plant and around the paint shop. As I'm going by, a lot of the people who work here will wave and smile like they're saying to themselves, "There's that crazy guy running again."

I can usually get in about four miles pretty easy during that 30 minutes. I'm not sure that the deadline to get back makes me faster, but it probably doesn't hurt. After production goes home, I'll go up to the fitness center and run on the treadmill for three to four more miles.

Since I really don't have time to change clothes, I wear my workout stuff underneath my coveralls. That way, as soon as I get outside, I can pull off them off and lay them beside the door and I'm gone. I also carry a pair of running shoes to work with me so that I can change into them before I go out to run. When I get back, I just put my coveralls on over my running stuff, dry myself off a little bit with a towel, and get back to work.

Since I use my breaks to run, I try to make time to eat on the job. So I bring stuff from home: things like apples, oranges, bananas, bagels, raisins, yogurt, and rice cakes. And about 99 percent of the time now, I drink water.

Sometimes they look at you funny when you're in a restaurant and order water to drink, but I'd rather have that than anything else. People are always asking me how I can stay so slim when I'm eating all the time. (I weigh about 165 pounds now.) You just have to stay active and eat the right kind of stuff.

My goal now is just to try to improve, to

get faster and win more races. To be a top seed in Atlanta's 10-K Peachtree Road Race you have to run under 36 minutes. For the past two years, I've qualified for the top group. And so far this year I've won two 10-Ks and one 5-K.

It's funny. I can remember looking at the Peachtree Road Race a few years back and they'd have 25,000 people running out there in all that heat, and I'd say that it looked like you would either get trampled to death or die of heatstroke. Now I wouldn't miss it for the world. At first, my friends couldn't believe that I was running either. But after your first 15 or 20 races, they're like, "What else is new?"

Part of History

I really hadn't thought about running the Boston Marathon too much until some of the guys at work said, "You ought to do it." Then I read some more about it, and I said, "Yeah, being the 100th anniversary I better go up and run in that." So I flew up there by myself.

About four or five hours before the start of the race, we were just lying around, just kind of there. And it's sort of cool, and I moved the wrong way or something and pulled something in my back. But I went ahead and ran the race.

It was a little slow starting with that big crowd—over 40,000 runners, including "bandits." But it was great. There were people lining the road almost the whole way, and they were hollering for you and giving you high fives and handing you water and fruit and stuff. It was exhilarating.

Everyone around me was running pretty hard—hard enough so that you couldn't really talk to anyone around you. And there were a lot of people in front of me, but I passed a lot of people, too.

After three hours and five minutes—and 26.2 miles—I crossed the finish line. The newspaper said that I came in 3,031. But when you think about it, it's kind of amazing that I was even there.

A Cut Above

Gary Israel, Fort Lauderdale, Florida

Date of birth: Oct. 9, 1958

Height and weight: 5-foot-11½, 168 pounds

Profession: Owner, men's Italian boutique

Sometimes when I'm running in the ocean along the beach at 5:00 A.M. and everything is so still and dark, I'll think back a few years. Back when I was so tired and in such pain that it was hard to face another day.

At the time, I was managing a men's clothing store company, helping them go from 3 South Florida stores to 22. It's an understatement to say that there was a lot of work and a lot of pressure. I did just about everything. Supervise the construction of the stores, inventory them, hire and train the employees, and even run the store for a time. It got to the point where I was working six and seven days a week from 7:30 A.M. until about 10:00 P.M. Obviously, there was no time to work out or do much of anything else. I was running myself ragged.

I was also eating anything and everything in sight. Hamburgers, pizza, whatever was convenient or in a mall, that's what I would have. A lot of sugar, too, just to keep going—especially desserts like chocolate cake and chocolate eclairs.

An Athletic Past

The only thing that I can think of that might have carried me through those seven years is my past history of athletics. I'm from South Africa originally, and when I was much younger I was involved in all kinds of sports: water skiing, diving, sailing, rugby, cricket. I came to the United States after graduating from high school and serving as a diver in the South African Navy. That's when I got involved in the men's clothing business, a business my family owned in South Africa as well.

By the time we were done with the expansion, I was very run down. My body was tired, and my feet ached. I ended up with a form of arthritis in my feet so bad that I could hardly walk. I went to all kinds of doctors, and some of them told me that I had to change my diet. One gave me medication that made my stomach burn.

Then one day, my father turned to me and said, "I can see that this isn't working. Get up in the mornings, go down to the beach, and I don't care if you can only do five steps, you have to start walking."

Well, I stopped the medication. And every morning I'd get up at 4:30, put on a pair of swimming trunks and a T-shirt, drive to the beach, and walk. And I'd try to walk a little further each morning. Week after week after week I went further and further and further. And that was really inspiring, because it started to work.

Getting a Lift

In the fall of 1994, a personal trainer named Bill Kyser came into my store. I could see that he was a very physically fit person, and we started talking. One thing led to another, and he agreed to train me. He's someone I wish I had met when I finished my military service, because at that time, there was nothing physical that I couldn't achieve. If I had a trainer or a coach like him around when I was younger, who knows where I could have gone.

Anyway, I had never lifted weights before, and Bill got me into a routine that involved training with weights—circuit training. Every Monday and Friday at 5:30 A.M., Bill comes over and puts me through the paces in a workshop in my house that I've partially converted into a mini-gym.

I start with a three-set per body part warm-up for my legs, shoulders and chest on a machine called the HydraFitness System (1-800-237-2271). The machine gives you resistance in both directions, and it lets you work all the major body parts. After you perform an overhead press to work your shoulders, you have to pull it back down, which works your back. It's the same thing after you do a leg extension; it turns into a leg curl that works your hamstrings. This machine is so advanced that the Navy has now incorporated it into its onboard submarine training program. No matter how sophisticated the equipment is, I make sure to warm up properly. It's a must ever since I injured my shoulder in a skiing accident a few years ago.

From there we go to bench presses: three sets of 15 with half a minute to a minute between sets. When we started I was using 90 pounds; now I'm pressing 185 pounds. Incline dumbbell presses are next for three or four sets with the same number of reps.

I used to hate training with weights. I didn't think you needed them. But inclines and dumbbell flies are my favorite exercises now. I've gone up in weight on my incline presses as well—from 25- to 55-pound dumbbells.

Next I do flies, chest pulls, lat pulls, shrugs, and chin-ups—three sets each. Then I go back to the HydraFitness system for two more sets: one performed faster with heavier weight and finally one burnout set of 20 reps for my chest, back, legs, and shoulders. We finish the circuit with three sets of curls and triceps presses.

To wrap up, I do three minutes of boxing, punching those pads that boxing trainers wear on their hands. I throw a lot of punches in those couple of minutes—jabs, upper cuts, even a little footwork. Normally, that's how we end the session, and by then, I'm ready to punch Bill. My arms feel like jelly, and I'm soaking wet. All in 1½ hours.

On Tuesday, Wednesday, and Thursday, I get up at the same time and go down to the beach for my hour run and walk in the water. I don't eat anything before I go, but I do drink four ounces of orange juice about 15 minutes beforehand. I start my beach routine with a fast walk to warm up, and then I'll run about three-quarters speed. Every half-mile or so along the way I'll stop and do 100 push-ups. When I get home, I do 20 chin-ups.

Before I started working with Bill, I weighed 158 pounds. Now I weigh 168 pounds. I've put on some muscle and lost some body fat. The first time Bill trained me, he asked me to do as many push-ups as I could in one minute. I did 83, which was a real surprise, given the shape I was in. Now I can easily do over 100 without stopping. I need to do more ab work, though, because I've neglected it.

In addition to my exercise routine, I'm now watching what I eat. I used to consume so much meat—steak, roasts, hamburgers. Now I eat meat about once a week.

Even with the changes I've made in my life, it's not always easy to fit a workout into my day. Six times a year I travel to Europe to buy clothing. It's usually a really tight schedule. For example, I'll fly out on Friday afternoon and return on either a Monday or Tuesday morning. Obviously, I don't have time for my normal workout routine, but I still do push-ups, and I walk an awful lot while I'm there. If there's a pool, I might go for a swim, but I don't lift weights when I'm away.

Because selling clothes is a very personalized business, people expect you to be there for them. Often that means working at night. Getting up as early as I do to exercise, you might think that I would need to get into bed earlier. But I usually don't turn in until between 11:00 P.M. and 11:30 P.M.

Still, it's worth it to work out in the morning because that allows me more time to spend with my wife, Beth, and sons, William and Zachary. If I waited until I came home from work to exercise, that would take time away from them. So it's a conscious effort on my part to say that I want to be healthy and I want to be fit but to do it early. And I'm prepared to make that sacrifice.

Mixing Bars and Barbells

John Schnupp, New York, New York

Date of birth: Nov. 29, 1963

Height and weight: 5-foot-7, 142 pounds

Profession: Restaurant manager

I grew up in a very competitive family. My dad always pushed athletics. But being in Manhattan made it different: We didn't play football with all the equipment; we played in the street. Hockey was on roller skates instead of ice skates. Basketball was the one true sport.

At age 14 or 15 I started reaching a level with bowling that I could never reach with other sports. It was just something that came very easy to me, so I stayed with it and kept progressing. Beginning at age 18, I spent about five years as a professional bowler.

There's not a lot of money in the game— not when I did it anyway. If you don't perform, you don't make anything. Meanwhile it costs money to enter tournaments, buy equipment, and travel. So you have to be good.

I never did as well as I should have. I'll always believe that I had the talent—I was just as good as any of them. But I was a single guy. Most of the guys on the tour have a wife and a child. They have to make money. Whereas I had a sponsor, so when I lost, it wasn't really my money. I wasn't as hungry as the other professionals. I was just happy to be out there.

Finally, my sponsor said, "I'm not supporting you anymore." That's when I got out.

Working Two Jobs

Now, I manage the bars at two restaurants. I started in this business when I was 13, and it's the only business I've ever known. Hopefully, I'll have the whole thing myself in two or three years. I think by the time I'm 35, I'll

be in a position to own my own place. I'm not talking about a four-star restaurant or anything, but I don't want just a little diner or luncheonette. That's not my goal.

I'll probably start out by opening a bar, because that doesn't require as much capital. If I can do that, then my plan is to put aside enough money that I can open a place I'll be really proud of. A two-star restaurant would be nice.

Right now, I obviously have to work hard to save some money. But the other part of it is all the time I'm investing in this business. I work 60 to 70 hours a week. And I learn. The person I learn from knows the restaurant business inside out—he was born into it. From watching him, I know how to stay on top of things, how to set things up so that they can almost run themselves.

The best part of my job is the interesting people I meet. We do have a lot of celebrities come in: John F. Kennedy, Jr.; Brad Pitt; Al Pacino; Matt Dillon. Michael Moriarty is a regular customer. There are times I get to know someone I can really connect with down the line.

Then there are the not-so-great things I deal with at work. I'll be honest with you, I hate having to make frozen drinks. It takes way too much time. Of course, this is the service industry. Some of the people you wait on aren't going to be satisfied no matter what you do for them. When something goes wrong, it takes a lot of effort to rectify the problem. It'll always cost you money, and the people you work for never want their money wasted. When I'm caught in the middle of a conflict like that, there's a lot of stress. I let it all out on the weights.

Working Out on the Late Shift

I get to work between 3:30 and 4:00 in the afternoon, six days a week. I'm there 9 to 11 hours. Sunday through Thursday I'm finished by around 1:30 A.M. Fridays and Saturdays tend to go later. I usually don't leave work until at least 2:30 A.M.

One of the restaurants where I work has a gym right above it open 24 hours on weekdays. So after we close and I've finished my paperwork for the night, I'll go upstairs to get in my workout, usually four times a week. I also go to the gym Saturday morning. I can't really spend six or seven days a week in the gym, because then I wouldn't have any energy left to do anything else. A good workout for me is 30 to 45 minutes. It can be that short because the gym is always empty. I don't have to wait to use the machines. I don't have any distractions—in a crowded gym, if I see a nice looking woman working out, my mind gets taken away.

Each night I go in, I try to do two sets of muscles that will work each other. I want to concentrate my workout as much as I can so that I can give my body time to recover. For instance, I start my week doing biceps and back—if I'm pulling on the rowing machine, my primary goal is to work my back, but I feel it in the biceps as well. That means that I don't have to spend as much time focused on my biceps, because they've already been working. I also work my abdominals every day. That goes without saying.

Tuesday I go for some cardiovascular training, but not too much, because I've been getting skinny. My metabolism is very high, and I just can't keep the weight on. Besides, I'm on my feet all day anyway. Running around back and forth on the job, you get a good workout.

Wednesday, I do chest and triceps. Thursday, shoulders and legs. Then I take Friday off. That night I work at the other restaurant, about 10 blocks from the gym, and I really don't want to walk over there at 2:30 in the morning. Saturday I go to the gym before work, probably getting in an extra workout on my back and biceps. Then Sunday I'm at the other restaurant, so I have that day off. That's my routine.

When I can't get to the gym, I still exercise. I'll do about 275 push-ups. I think they're

the best exercise to work the most amount of muscle groups. I get a pretty complete workout with that—back, chest, triceps, shoulders.

After I work out at the gym, most of the time I can go out with someone for a while and still get home by 4:00 A.M. So I read the morning paper, am in bed by 5:00 A.M. and get my seven to eight hours sleep.

A Religious Experience

I think everyone wants to look good and feel good. You just have to decide whether you'll work hard for it. You need something to get you going. I joined the gym at the beginning of February, and about two weeks later I gave up drinking for Lent. That's when I seriously got into the weights and my diet. I decided that I didn't have any more excuses. If I could change my routine for Lent, I could change it for good. I pretty much gave up red meat and dairy. I'm very rigid about it. I have a lot of pasta, tuna, fresh turkey, some chicken, vegetables, and lots of fruit.

I've seen a lot of people who work out four or five times a week, but they eat whatever they want, so there's no real result. All they're doing is putting some mass on top of whatever fat they have. They get bigger, but they don't really look good. That's not what I wanted.

It's not easy. It takes a lot of discipline. But this is what I have to do, and I accept that. I will stand in front of the mirror and tell myself, "If you expect to keep this body, then you're not going to eat ice cream or you're not going to skip this workout." And I've lost about 15 pounds since I started.

My social life has picked up a bit—which I wasn't even really looking for. I'm more confident in myself, to the point of sometimes being a little cocky. When you've toned your body up, you want people to look at it, to see how hard you worked. It makes me feel good to know that I'm probably in better shape than 90 percent of the men my age.

Fighting for Fitness

Louis Lanza, New York, New York

Date of birth: Nov. 30, 1961

Height and weight: 5-foot-6, 158 pounds

Profession: Restaurant owner and chef

I didn't start as a physically promising specimen. I was born with a double hernia. The doctors had to operate on me at the age of six weeks.

When I was five, my parents dropped me in the water, and I've been swimming ever since. I swam competitively from age 6 to 18. My specialties were the 50- and the 100-yard freestyle events. Swimming is great for every part of your body, especially the upper body. And it's a great low-impact aerobic workout. It was the foundation for all the high school sports I competed in. As a running back in football, for example, it was very hard to pull me down. And I always had incredible stamina thanks to swimming. I once ran a marathon with only two days' training.

You could say that I short-circuited my way into the restaurant business. Originally, I had planned to become an electrical engineer, but after a year of school it turned out that I hated engineering. Inspired by my Sicilian grandmother, who first taught me a love of cooking and the importance of using fresh ingredients, I entered a two-year program in hotel and restaurant management. I've been working in restaurants ever since.

To honor my grandmother, I named two of my Manhattan restaurants after her: Josephina, across from Lincoln Center, and Josie's Restaurant and Juice Bar, on the Upper West Side. Sometimes I work several hours at Josephina, serving 200 dinners to the pre-theater crowd in a span of two hours, then I run uptown to Josie's and Ansonia (another restaurant of mine) for the remainder of the night.

Most chefs work 15-hour days. It's exhausting. Now I wear three hats: I'm an owner, a general manager, and the executive chef of Josie's. Talk about pressure. Talk about stress. Here's one week in my life. One morning a cook calls in sick. Who do you think fills in? Me. Another day the local striped bass I planned to use look bad. I have to quickly come up with something else before we print the day's menu. One evening I find out that we've overbooked the dining room, and I'm praying that there are some no-shows. The next night we have a bunch of cancellations, and I'm praying for some walk-in traffic. The ceiling is leaking. I'm not getting along with my partner. Mind you, this is all in the same week.

In This Corner: Mr. Mellow

When I was younger I would lose my temper easily. The kitchen is a very intense place to work. It's hot, it's crowded, and there are deadlines every second. I had a very short fuse. I took everything so seriously. I worked like a dog. I'd build up a lot of aggression and blow up at waiters in the kitchen. Now that I'm out on the dining room floor, I can't let my emotions out.

Boxing is my savior. I go into the gym, start hitting the bag, and break a sweat, and the stress and strain start to melt away. After a couple rounds of sparring, you have no desire to be a maniac in the kitchen. I discovered boxing in 1994. I had been into martial arts when I was younger. But I wasn't very flexible and had trouble with it.

Since that first hernia, I've had two others. Boxing doesn't require that kind of flexibility. Also, I was impatient. Martial arts requires lots of training. With boxing you can get into it faster. There's more immediate gratification. When I get into something, I like to do it right away.

Plus, it's unbelievable the shape that you have to be in to box. And it's like an art.

Despite the image of the dumb boxer, it's a thinking man's sport. You're bobbing in and out, ducking, and weaving. You need quick hand-eye coordination, always thinking about when to attack and when to back off.

As for how I fit working out in, I'm usually up at 9:00 A.M. The first thing I do is go to the restaurant and spend a couple hours or so doing administrative work. Then I go into the kitchen for another hour or so, setting up and prepping for the day. At about noon I'll go to the gym. I try to get to the gym three or four times a week.

I warm up for a half-hour. I stretch for 10 minutes, combining yoga with other stretching. I do sit-ups on a big rubber ball. I throw the 20-pound medicine ball and do a series of chin-ups and dips—about 8 to 10 sets. Then I cross-train, one day running on the treadmill, the next riding a bicycle machine.

Another day I jump rope: front, crossing, one leg, two legs. Then I hit the bags for a half-hour, first the heavy bag, then the speed bag. I do 7 to 10 three-minute rounds, with a minute interval. In between I do push-ups. On other days I'll spar for 6 to 8 three-minute rounds, with a minute between. I'll finish off with some bag work and shadowboxing.

Now I'm into another sport: surfing. I used to bodysurf as a kid. But now I've taken it up with a vengeance. I go out to Long Island on weekends. I've even hired a pro to teach me. Talk about a sport to get you in shape! The exercise is not riding the waves; it's paddling out to the waves. It's a total upper-body workout. I come home with sore shoulders.

Recipe for Health

The other important part of staying healthy, of course, is how you eat and how you deal with illness when you do get sick. I believe in using natural foods and alternative methods of medicine. The thing that sold me on this was when my girlfriend at the time was diagnosed with a thyroid tumor. Doctors recommended surgery, but I thought that there must be an alternative.

She went to a chiropractor who took a holistic approach. For one thing, he recommended that she change her diet. Together we got into macrobiotics, a diet that excludes dairy and meat and emphasizes lots of fresh seasonal organic vegetables and grains. This was hard for me because I was a real dairy-lover. Eventually, my girlfriend's thyroid shrank so much that surgery was unnecessary. For me, my body fat took a dramatic drop. When I saw how my whole body changed, I knew this was powerful stuff.

That diet influenced me so much that when I opened Josie's, I concentrated on organically grown produce. There's no dairy, preservatives, or concentrated fats in our dishes. Even the water we use for drinking, cooking, and ice cubes is triple-filtered to remove chlorine, fluoride, and harmful bacteria.

At the juice bar we serve fresh-squeezed juice and vegetable drinks, spiked with fresh ginger, aloe vera, and bee pollen. Though I eat meat from time to time and we serve it in the restaurant, I buy and eat only free-range meats. That means that the foods that the animals eat are whole grains and that they are allotted a certain amount of free-running space. I don't think that meat is bad; what's bad is what the animals are fed and injected with (antibiotics, growth hormones, appetite stimulants), which often contains steroids and other chemicals.

But don't get me wrong. I'm not adamant about things. I believe in moderation. Italian food with a tiramisu dessert is fine every once in awhile.

My basic philosophy is this: If I can get to the halfway point in whatever I'm doing, I can see the finish line. And knowing how satisfied I'll be when I get there is all I need to motivate me to keep pushing. Halfway is my watershed. The rest is downhill.

To Live and Work Out in L.A.

Scott Devine, Sherman Oaks, California

Date of birth: Mar. 14, 1969

Height and weight: 6 feet, 215 pounds

Profession: Agent's assistant

When I was in college, I was like 95 percent of the guys in the gym: I wanted to be as big as possible. But with the job I have now—an assistant at International Creative Management (ICM), one of the largest talent agencies in the world—just staying in shape is a challenge.

I had always dreamed about going to Los Angeles. Before I made the jump, though, I figured that I should check it out. So I flew out there from Milwaukee and looked around for a week or so and said, "Yeah, I'm definitely going to give this a try."

I went home and told my parents about what I wanted to do. They said, "Great. When do you think you'll go?" And I said, "Monday." Within a week, I literally packed everything into my car and drove the 2,300 miles by myself to give it a shot.

Act I: The Kid's Big Break

I don't have any uncles in the movie business or anything, so I wasn't quite sure what I was going to do. Then a friend of mine told me about a temp agency that specialized in the film industry. After I hooked up with them, one day the phone rang, and they asked whether I'd be willing to work in the mail room at ICM.

I had heard stories about agents and other people getting their start in the mail room of a talent agency, so I swallowed my pride and my master's degree in film and video production and went to work. I guess they liked me, because they asked me to stick around. After spending two months as a floating assistant, I landed a permanent job as assistant to Jack Gilardi, one of the company's executive vice-presidents and a legend in the agency business.

Working as an agent in Hollywood isn't just hanging around smoking cigars, drinking cognac, and schmoozing. Agents work hard to help put together the deals that help actors, directors, and writers—what's called above-the-line talent—get jobs in movies. But it's a tricky situation. Sometimes the buyers—producers and studios—complain that we ask for too much. Sometimes our clients—actors, screenwriters, and directors—complain because they think that we aren't asking enough. As you might imagine, this can be fairly stressful. You have to be part businessman, part diplomat, and part psychiatrist.

And even after you help someone get a job, that's not the end of the story. Nearly everyone in Hollywood is, in essence, a freelancer or a temp. You help get an actor a job on a film; they're working for six weeks, two months, six months tops; and then they're looking for another job.

If there isn't anything waiting for them at the end of that project, they're naturally a little cranky. It's like "Okay, this person has something for now, but they're going to need something else real soon." And if you have 15 to 20 clients—many agents have more—it makes for a lot of work.

My boss takes a lot of meetings, and while he's gone I have to hold down the fort. Just because he's out doesn't mean that the work stops. In fact, it seems like when he leaves, the phone calls roll in. We handle 120 to 150 phone calls a day—easy. I'm on the phone so much sometimes that I think I have one permanently attached to my head.

I also read film scripts and write what is called coverage for ICM. Coverage is a fancy name for a book report that describes the script and whether it reads like it would make a good movie. Does the story work? Are the characters interesting and unique?

Sometimes people will ask me about the best part of a particular script. More often than not, I'll say the fact that it was only 90 pages long. There are a lot of really bad scripts out there. On the other hand, there are times when I'm working and we get a hot script, and it's like "Drop everything—we need some coverage in two hours."

Act II: Scott's Hollywood Workout

Needless to say, I don't have a lot of extra time, so if I'm going to get in a workout, I have to first win the battle with the snooze button on my alarm clock. Back in college when I had all the time in the world, I would loosen up for 15 to 20 minutes on a bike or treadmill—anything to get the blood flowing—and then slap the weights around.

It was lift hard and see how much can you do. The gyms I went to were pretty hardcore, and even though I had a decent build, I was still one of the smaller guys there. There were bouncers, professional wrestlers, and even a guy who would finish high in the Mr. America competition. It was great motivation.

From the time I walk into the gym at 7:00 A.M. to the time I walk out, I give myself an hour. I don't take long breaks between sets and exercises. Because I know that I can work out faster and don't like waiting for the machines, I prefer to be in the gym when it's empty.

Some people do a set and sit there for 1½ minutes—their workout will take 1½ hours when they're only doing 45 minutes of work. My thing is to do the set, put down the weight for no more than 15 seconds, catch my breath, look at the clock and then go to the next set. When I'm done, boom, wipe the machine down and then go to the next one knowing how much weight I'll use, how to set it up, and then go right into it. It's more like circuit training.

I'm also doing a lot more of the machines than free weights now. So I'll do the chest press, then the pec deck, the lat pull-down, and the triceps machine and just go right down the line.

And I don't even train my legs anymore. I've always had big legs from playing soccer, so I figure when I'm doing my cardiovascular work to warm up like biking or the treadmill, that works my legs. And then on the weekend when I try to do some fun stuff like in-line skating, biking, hiking, or something like that, I know that my legs are getting a good workout.

Act III: Eating on the Run

I don't work through lunch too often. If I need to catch up on something, I grab a quick bite, but I like my lunch hour and use it. It's a chance for me to get out of the building, usually somewhere in Beverly Hills. And you need an hour for lunch here. If you go out anywhere, with the driving, the parking, and all that, it's an hour—easy.

I know some people who blow off lunch. But if you're going nonstop from the start of the day to the end with no break, it can really wear you down. Burnout is common in talent agencies.

After working until 7:00 P.M. and commuting for 45 minutes back into the valley, the last thing I want to do is think about what I can have for dinner. So when I go shopping, I try to plan what I'm going to eat for the next week. When I went to the store the other day, I knew that I had some leftover ground turkey in the fridge, so I decided that I'd make a turkey meat loaf that will last me two days, grab some salmon for Wednesday, and for a vegetarian day or two, pick up some spaghetti and mushrooms and salad. That way I'm not wasting time going to the grocery store three or four times a week.

I won't do this forever, but until I can write and sell my own script, I'm learning a lot—especially about how to manage my time.

Male Makeovers Finding the time for exercise—and getting the most out of it when you do—isn't easy. So we turned to the experts for their best advice for some common scenarios. See if any sound familiar.

His Health Is on the Line

The Scenario

Tom is 26 years old, newly married, and slightly overweight. A varsity wrestler during his high school years, Tom never had to worry about his health and fitness—until lately. He thought that his job on a machine-parts assembly line would keep him in shape. It's hard work, involving a lot of heavy lifting that has equipped him with bulging biceps. The only problem is that he has acquired a bulging belly as well.

His diet is heavy on bar grub—nachos, chicken wings, subs, and, of course, beer—and fast-food burgers. Working a rotating shift, Tom rarely finds time for exercise, even the basketball and football games that he loves to play with his buddies, and there are weeks he barely sees his wife.

The Solution

My first thought after reading Tom's profile was, how did he keep from becoming the Good Year blimp? So many people confuse manual labor with aerobic or cardiovascular exercise. Tom's work on the assembly line is not doing his new belly much good. Games of football and basketball are fun and certainly a way of moving, which is beneficial, but they are not fat-burning. To burn fat, and to lose approximately one pound a week, there needs to be continuous movement for at least 20 minutes (it actually takes 20 minutes to start burning fat), and it should be done four or five times a week.

Since Tom's hours are odd and he and his wife have trouble finding time together, I suggest that Tom invest in a stair-climber. It is an effective way to burn fat, work leg muscles, and still provide an opportunity for him to spend time with his wife or catch up on a show or two. He'll also find a surge of energy after the workout. Also, Tom shouldn't be afraid to integrate rope jumping into his cardiovascular routine to keep his heart pumping. I would suggest spending less time in the bars. Instead, try socializing more as couples. Remember, in people's homes, low-fat snacks are easier and more accessible to make. Tom's diet is very high in fat and low in nutrition. With today's choices being so much wider, Tom can avoid the high-fat burgers and fries and instead choose a grilled chicken sandwich and salad.

While I wouldn't ask Tom to give up snacks, I would suggest that he stick to items like pretzels and fruit. If he can keep his own stash of snacks, this will prevent him from the temptation once he's there. Plus, if you spend $15 a week in the snack room, that adds up to more than $700 a year that could be put toward vacation time with his wife. I recommend that Tom keep the football and basketball games—they're great for the spirit—but bring bottled water. Rather than thinking of these changes as a diet or form of deprivation, think of it as improving and investing in a healthy lifestyle.

—Marc Goodman, fitness instructor and personal trainer at Crunch, a gym in New York City

Enjoying the Good Things in Life

The Scenario

Life as a traveling computer consultant has many perks and just as many unhealthy drawbacks. Brian spends most of his time in big cities, foreign and domestic ports, dining in the best restaurants, staying at the finest hotels, and—if he can get a break from the seemingly endless round of meetings—slipping out for some sight-seeing. Brian has spent most of his 50-odd years working hard to reach this point, and he fully intends to enjoy it.

His children are grown, his wife is happily retired, and all should be well. Yet Brian is somewhat unhappy with his physique. He doesn't expect to look like he did when he was 20 (or even 30), but he knows that he should lose a few pounds. His wife has taken up speed walking and encourages him to tag along, but after one neighborhood block he is out of breath and ready to call a taxi for the trip home. He would like to have the same energy for his grandchildren as he did for his kids 25 years ago.

Brian's not sure how age has crept up on him. He has a fondness for scotch and good cigars on occasion and thoroughly enjoys the five-course meals on his business trips. He figures that he can make up for his indulgences with a few laps in the hotel pool, followed by a relaxing session in the sauna.

The Solution

Brian can get back in shape if he is persistent about it. He needs to set a goal to get a cardiovascular workout three times a week for 30 to 45 minutes. The first thing he should do is visit his family doctor for a complete physical before he begins any regular exercise routine. This is important not only because of his age but also because he can get some personalized exercise advice.

My next suggestion would be to invest in a basic heart monitor—you can get them at most bike or fitness stores for about $100. Of all the different measures for physical fitness, this is the most accessible and gives an instant biofeedback measure. Heart monitors are easy to operate. You simply strap it around your chest and put on the watch and away you go. Brian's heart rate will be directly measured, and he will be able to notice the threshold of when calories are burned. It is a good way to determine workout intensity and will also monitor recovery time. Brian's heart rate should fall beneath 100 beats per minute within five minutes of ending an exercise. The more you observe your heart, the more you might get interested in your body.

I would suggest a treadmill for the most effective way to burn fat, and he can even watch CNN. On business trips Brian should opt to skip the taxi and go it on foot. Swimming laps is a good idea, too. It offers strength-training benefits because of the water resistance.

Brian's large meals contribute to weight gain and leave less energy after eating. He should eat more frequent and smaller meals and have healthy snacks that will give him more energy to live life.

—Joe Ogilvie, fitness leader at Chelsea Piers Sports and Entertainment Center in New York City

Stuck on the Business Treadmill

The Scenario

Kevin is an advertising executive at a big agency in New York City. In his mid-thirties and unmarried, he thinks about and does little else than hustle for his next ad account. On average, he puts in 12-hour days, which often include meetings that run through lunch and late-night business dinners. Considering that he never eats breakfast, Kevin's diet consists mainly of snacks from the vending machines at work, very heavy late-evening dinners with his clients, and lots and lots of coffee.

He's also a smoker, puffing on at least a pack a day. Taking cabs all over the city and always opting for the elevator instead of the stairs, Kevin never really notices the toll that the cigarettes and the inactivity are exacting on his body until he tries to play a round of golf or a set of tennis.

The Solution

Heredity and lifestyle are the two leading contributors of health risks. Kevin's lifestyle has all the ingredients of poor health—unfavorable eating patterns, sedentary habits, smoking, and stress. These four factors point to present and future problems. The good news is that Kevin can make some changes.

In order to improve his fitness level, Kevin needs to try to exercise four or five times a week. Since Kevin works 12-hour days, he needs several exercise plans to accommodate his hectic professional schedule. One option would be to choose a gym near his home or office so that it is very convenient to get to. As for scheduling his visits to the gym, Kevin should try for an hour on one early morning before work, one lunch hour during the week, and then one hour on Saturday and one on Sunday. This way, Kevin can adapt his workout schedule to his work schedule with a lot of flexibility and options.

Weeks when Kevin can't fit one-hour exercise programs into his schedule shouldn't deter him. During such hectic weeks, Kevin should try to work in exercise throughout his days. Maybe he could have the taxi let him off 5 to 10 blocks before his destinations, or he could decide to always take the stairs instead of the elevator. A third option for Kevin would be to get up 15 minutes earlier and walk briskly toward the office. After 15 minutes, grab a cab for the remainder of the trip. Kevin needs to keep in mind that some exercise is better than nothing, and since he is already overwhelmed by his job, he shouldn't feel overwhelmed by his workouts. Regular exercise might also help Kevin to kick the cigarette habit, since he may voluntarily want to cut down on the smoking as he starts to feel better about himself.

Improving his eating habits is another positive change that Kevin needs to consider. Kevin's long days and nights require food choices that are high in nutrition. If he knows that a meeting is likely to run through lunch, Kevin should arrange with a local deli or restaurant to have his lunch delivered to his office so that he can dig in right after the meeting. Late-night dinners should be lighter, so Kevin needs to plan ahead again and have a larger lunch on those days. In general, Kevin needs to learn to balance his life and make an effort to eat, live, and work healthier so that the rest of his years can be productive and energetic.

—Courtney Barroll, certified personal trainer and medical exercise specialist at Equinox Fitness Club in New York City

His Dilemma: Family or Fitness?

The Scenario

A senior computer analyst by day and a devoted father and husband by night, Matthew crams a lot into 24 hours. A typical workday begins with a hearty breakfast à la Joyce (Matthew's wife). Well-fed and with his brown-bag lunch in hand, Matthew takes to the highway, where he will spend the next 60 minutes battling the rush-hour commute from the suburbs into the city. After nine hours of sitting chained to his computer terminal, Matthew again finds himself sitting behind the wheel of his sport utility vehicle, hoping that his 60-minute return commute doesn't turn into a 90-minute nightmare as a result of a jackknifed tractor trailer.

Feeling guilty that he spends so much time away from his children, Matthew reserves most of his evenings for escorting his two sons to their karate lessons and soccer games. He would love to devote a little time to his own physical fitness—about the only time he gets out now is for the occasional skiing trip that he takes during the winter months—but he just doesn't see how he can squeeze in his own workout without compromising the little bit of time he spends with his family.

The Solution

Matthew has to realize that working some exercise into his daily life will benefit both him and his family. Regular workouts will help give Matthew more energy throughout the day, keep him more focused at work, and make his life, in general, more productive.

Incorporating exercise into his already-packed day will be much easier for Matthew if he has some type of support group to encourage him and keep him motivated. In Matthew's case, his family seems to be the most logical and convenient answer. Having two young sons that he wants to spend more time with anyway, Matthew can plan some of his exercise time with the kids. He could set up a basketball net outside the house and play some one-on-one a couple nights a week. Chances are that Matthew's kids will really look forward to the games with their dad and keep Matthew faithful to his scheduled family basketball nights.

Maybe Matthew also could join in during his sons' karate lessons or jog around the soccer field a few times instead of standing around during the kids' soccer practices. On weekends, Matthew can take the initiative and plan some family outings that are centered around active pursuits such as hiking, biking, or swimming. All these changes will allow Matthew to get some exercise while also spending good quality time with his children.

Matthew's wife, Joyce, can help support him in his decision to work more exercise into his workday by changing their present morning ritual of early-morning talks over massive breakfasts to vigorous conversation during a 30-minute brisk walk around the neighborhood. As the two of them become more fit through their new morning regimen, both will most likely become more conscious about their current eating habits and make some subtle changes that can make a big nutrition difference.

—Rebecca Gorrell, certified exercise leader and wellness education director at Canyon Ranch Fitness Resort in Tucson, Arizona

Fumbling Away His Fitness

The Scenario

Nate has always been a physically imposing guy. In high school, he lived in the weight room and on the football field. Now in his early twenties, he works construction for eight hours and then heads over to the local gym for another hour of lifting.

Unfortunately, he doesn't seem to be getting much out of his lifting program anymore. For one thing, he doesn't have the football coach standing over him barking out orders and making him hit the track as well as the weights. In his mind, running is something that you do for punishment when you screw up. There are also a lot more interesting women at the gym than there were at his football practices.

Nate gets most of his nutrition advice from his weight-lifting buddies. As a result, his daily diet includes lots of supplements, energy bars, and high-protein drinks. Nate believes that he can still get away with eating more than the average guy because of his physically demanding job and his regular weight-training program. Yet recently, Nate has noticed that his muscle tone seems to be fading beneath a softer, fleshier layer.

The Solution

Since Nate hasn't been playing football for a few years now, he needs to start thinking about a more general, health-related training program with some new short-term goals. These goals should be things that can be achieved fairly easily to keep Nate's motivation level high so that he will continue and strive for the longer-term goals. Maybe Nate can try a new sport that he's always wanted to play and then build a new workout program around the basic skills and demands of this new sport. Or perhaps he would want to try his hand at a number of new sports, with his ultimate goal being participation in a biathlon or triathlon.

Nate's new exercise program needs to include some aerobic training. While Nate uses his muscles all day on the construction site, he is doing very little for his cardiovascular fitness and, therefore, needs to balance his strength training with aerobic activities. Once again, Nate needs to get past the mentality of his football days, when running was the coach's main form of punishment. Whether it's biking, jogging, or using the stair-climbers at the gym that he frequents, Nate should be shooting for 30 to 45 minutes of aerobic training from three to five times a week. A good goal for Nate would be to try not to go more than two days in a row without some type of aerobic exercise. Maybe Nate could ask one of those interesting women at the gym if they wanted to join him for a jog on side-by-side treadmills.

Just as Nate's exercise program reflects his days as a football player, so does his diet. All those supplements, energy bars, and protein drinks may have been helpful to Nate back in high school, but now they seem to be fueling him with too many unnecessary calories. Adding the aerobic training to his workout schedule will help to burn some of those calories, but Nate should concentrate on eating more real foods in the form of a balanced diet.

—Steven Wheelock, fitness co-director of Canyon Ranch Lifestyle Resort in Lenox, Massachusetts

Index

Note: Underscored page references indicate boxed text or photographs. **Boldface** page references indicate main discussion of topic.

Devine, Scott, 156–57
Israel, Gary, 150–51
Lanza, Louis, 154–55
O'Brien, Pat, 136–37, <u>136</u>
Peters, Tom, 146–47, <u>146</u>
Schnupp, John, 152–53
Recovery from workout, 9
Relaxation exercises, <u>133</u>
Relaxation response, 88
Rempel, David, 106–7
Resistance training, 49
Rest between workouts, 23, 32
Reverse crunch exercise, 45, <u>45</u>
Rippe, James M., 2–3
Road biking. *See* Bicycling
Roberts, Scott, <u>78</u>
Roberts, Susan, 96
Robinson, John P., 3
Rodgers, Marge, <u>89</u>, 106–7
Rollers, 63
Rowing machine, <u>15</u>
Rudow, Martin, 77, <u>77</u>
Running, **68–69**
  aerobic exercise and, 67
  benefits of, 68
  calories burned by, 48
  cross-training for, <u>69</u>
  deep-water, <u>73</u>
  in fat-burning workout, 49
  with hand weights, 17
  hill training for, 69, <u>73</u>
  scheduling time for, 68
  sprinting, 68–69, <u>75</u>, 103
  techniques, 68–69
  10-K, 21–22
  before tennis, 74–75
  uphill, 69, <u>73</u>
Ruppel, Howard, Jr., 113

S

Salad, 103
Salt, 103
Saviano, Nick, 74–75, <u>75</u>
Scheduling time for exercise,
  2–3, 68, **80–83**, <u>82–83</u>

Schinfeld, Jay S., 27
Schnueringer, Elaine, 4
Schnupp, John, 152–53
Scott, Steve, <u>65</u>, 68–69
Seated dumbbell curls, 38, <u>38</u>
Seated military press, 38, <u>38</u>
Seated overhead triceps
  extension, 38, <u>38</u>
Seated row, 134
Seated side bend, 46, <u>46</u>
Seated two-arm row, 41, <u>41</u>
  with tubing, 55
Self-massage, <u>133</u>
Self-test for health and fitness, 5
Sex, **26–27**, <u>27</u>, 80
Shoulder and wrist stretch, 95, <u>95</u>
Shoulder press, 99, <u>99</u>
Shoulder shrug, 88, 94, <u>94</u>
Showering after workouts, 86,
  130–31, <u>131</u>
Side oblique crunch exercise, 45,
  <u>45</u>
Singer, Judy, 104–5
60-minute workout, **56–57**,
  <u>56–57</u>
Skiing, **70–71**, <u>71</u>
Sleep, 30, 109
Sleeping pills, 80
Slide board, horizontal, <u>67</u>
Smith, Kathy, 15
Smoking, quitting, 20
Snacks, 100, 105
Soap, antibacterial, 130
Social workout, **112–13**, <u>113</u>
Soda, 121. *See also* Caffeine
Sodium, 103
Soileau, Michael, 16
Solis, Ken, 132
Soreness, muscle, 7, 64–65, 71
Soup, 103, <u>125</u>
Speed golf, <u>65</u>
Spence, Steve, 68–69, <u>69</u>
Spinning class, 63
Split step, 75
Spohn, Don, 106
Sports. *See specific types*

Sprinting, 68–69, <u>75</u>, 103
Squat, 43, <u>43</u>, 57, 71
S-shaped pull, 73
Stair climbing, 93, 105
Stamford, Bryant, 68, 114
Stationary bike, 63
Stephens, "Spanky," 72–73
Stern, Doug, <u>73</u>
Steroids, 9
Stiff-legged dead lift, 39, <u>39</u>
Stone, Michael, 12
Storzo, Gary A., 104
Strength training, **11–13**, <u>12–13</u>,
  15–16, 73, 134. *See also*
    Weight lifting
Stress, 80, <u>89</u>
Stretching, **18–19**, **94–95**
  for basketball, 61
  before chores, 115
  before exercise, general,
    18–19, <u>19</u>
  on fence, 88
  flexibility and, 18–19
  for golf, 65
  muscle, 19
  office, 94–95, <u>94–95</u>
  techniques, correct, 18–19
  at work, <u>19</u>
Substitutes for specific exercises,
  <u>117</u>
Supersets, <u>9</u>
Supper, 30, 103, 127
Sweat, <u>27</u>, 130, <u>131</u>
Swimming, 22–23, **72–73**, <u>73</u>
Swing-shift workout, **108–9**

T

Tea, 121. *See also* Caffeine
Television shows, exercise,
  105
10-K run, 21–22
10-minute ab workout, **44–47**,
  <u>44–47</u>
10-minute workout, **50**, <u>50</u>
Tennis, **74–75**, <u>75</u>